Managing Pain in the Older Adult

Michaelene P. Jansen, RN, C, PhD, GNP-BC, FNP, C is a professor of nursing in the College of Nursing and Health Sciences at the University of Wisconsin–Eau Claire. She is a certified family and gerontological nurse practitioner and is certified by the American Nurses Credentialing Center in Pain. She has worked with chronic pain patients at the Pain Clinic of Northwestern Wisconsin for many years. Her professional career includes advanced practice nursing in primary care, pain, and pulmonary clinics. Professional nurse experiences include critical care and trauma. She has coedited three editions of *Advanced Practice Nursing, Core Concepts for Professional Role Development,* published by Springer Publishing.

Managing Pain in the Older Adult

Michaelene P. Jansen, RN, C, PhD, GNP-BC, FNP, C

EDITOR

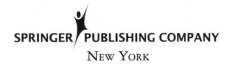

SPRINGER PUBLISHING COMPANY

NEW YORK

Springer Publishing Company, LLC
11 West 42nd Street
New York, NY 10036
www.springerpub.com

Acquisitions Editor: Allan Graubard
Production Editor: Julia Rosen
Cover design: Joanne E. Honigman
Composition: Apex Publishing, LLC

08   09   10/   5   4   3   2   1

Library of Congress Cataloging-in-Publication Data

Managing pain in the older adult / [edited by] Michaelene P. Jansen.
     p. ; cm.
   Includes bibliographical references and index.
   ISBN 978-0-8261-1567-6 (alk. paper)
  1. Pain in old age—Treatment.   I. Mirr Jansen, Michaelene P.
  [DNLM: 1. Pain—therapy.   2. Aged.   3. Combined Modality Therapy. WL 704 M2667 2008]

   RB127.M347   2008
   618.97'60472—dc22

                                    2007051942

Printed in the United States of America by Bang Printing.

This book is dedicated to the special men in my life, Mark, Brian, Paul, Kirk, and Keil. Their love and support is deeply appreciated.
MPJ

Contents

Contributors

Kerri M. Crank, RN, MSN, FNP-BC, CNRN
Family Nurse Practitioner
Department of Neurology
Luther Midelfort
Eau Claire, Wisconsin

Karen S. Feldt, RN, PhD, GNP-BC
Associate Professor, Seattle
University College of Nursing
Gerontological Nurse Practitioner
Northwest Geriatrics
Mercer Island, Washington

Amanda Gentilli
University of Wisconsin–Eau Claire
Eau Claire, Wisconsin

Ann Hoepner, RN, C, BSN
Implant Coordinator
Pain Clinic of Northwestern
Wisconsin
Eau Claire, Wisconsin

Michele Komp-Webb, DPT
Department of Physical Therapy
Luther Hospital
Eau Claire, Wisconsin

Susan D. Peck, RN, PHD, GNP-BC, CHTP
Professor, Gerontological Nurse
Practitioner
University of Wisconsin–Eau Claire
Eau Claire, Wisconsin

Melissa M. Tomesh, RN, MSN
Instructor
Chippewa Valley Technical College
Eau Claire, Wisconsin

Preface

The older adult population is the fastest-growing segment of our society. It is estimated that by 2030, 22% of the population will be over 65 years of age. The majority of that population will have at least one chronic health condition. Over 70% will experience some form of persistent pain. The challenge for health care providers is to understand the mechanisms of acute and chronic pain as well as the physiologic changes associated with aging.

Although our knowledge of aging and pain continues to grow daily, both continue to challenge health care providers. The older population poses unique health care issues and challenges. Persistent pain is under-recognized and under-treated. Providers are often hesitant to treat pain in older adults due to adverse effects and interactions of many of the treatment options. A deeper understanding of common pain syndromes and treatments for older adults will provide a more comprehensive approach to their persistent pain.

This text is written as a reference for health care providers seeking to expand their knowledge of pain in the older population. The intent of the book is to provide a user-friendly approach to examine various treatment options as well as some of the cautions that need to be heeded in treating pain in the older population. The better the understanding of pain in older cognitive and cognitively impaired adults will result in better pain control for this population.

The book is organized in two sections. The first section explores background information on pain in the elderly and common pain syndromes. Special consideration for assessing pain and pain-related behaviors in the older population is included in this section. A chapter related to sleep and behavioral aspects of pain in older adults provides insight into environmental influences on pain and pain perception.

The second section of this book is dedicated to the management of pain in the elderly. A multimodality approach to pain management is emphasized. Most chronic conditions, pain being no exception, are best treated with multiple therapies, as one method of treatment is limiting. The chapters on physical therapy, interventions, and complementary therapies provide alternatives for older adults in managing their pain. Special considerations for use of pharmacotherapeutic agents with older adults are provided in a separate chapter. Improving mobility and function in patients with persistent pain is the focus of another chapter.

Managing Pain in the Older Adult is unique in that the focus of the text centers specifically on the needs of the older person suffering from pain. Improving function and quality of life are priorities in treating this population. This text is targeted toward primary care providers, as they are the health professionals that older adults feel most comfortable with in discussing their health concerns. Early recognition of pain syndromes in the elderly can lead to earlier treatment and control of pain, thus decreasing the development of undesired pain-related behaviors or co-morbidities.

Michaelene P. Jansen

Acknowledgments

I would like to acknowledge the help and support of several individuals and institutions in the development of this text. The patients and staff at the Pain Clinic of Northwestern Wisconsin have been instrumental in helping me understand the mechanisms involved in the transmission of pain and the effects that pain has in the lives of those affected. I would also like to acknowledge the support of the University of Wisconsin–Eau Claire and Office of Research and Sponsored Programs in the development and writing of this manuscript.

SECTION I

Background Information

CHAPTER 1

Pain in Older Adults

Michaelene P. Jansen

Pain has been defined by the International Association for the Study of Pain as an unpleasant sensory and emotional experience associated with potential or actual tissue damage. This is the most widely used definition when describing the concept of pain. Pain accompanies many health conditions across all ages and presents a challenge for health care providers. Pain can be acute or chronic in nature. Pain is considered persistent or chronic if it occurs for three or more months. The American Geriatric Society (AGS) adopted the term *persistent pain* in lieu of chronic pain to promote a more positive perception of ongoing pain. Table 1.1 describes attributes associated with acute and persistent pain. The purpose of this text, and particularly this chapter, is to explore the concept of pain and its unique characteristics in the older population.

The older adult population is the fastest-growing segment in our society. Approximately 36 million Americans, or 12% of the population, are over 65 years of age (Federal Interagency Forum on Age-Related Statistics, 2004). Between 2010 and 2030, the older adult population is expected to grow by 75% to over 69 million. The greatest increase will be seen in the over-85-year-old population. It is estimated that the over-85-year-old population will increase to 18.2 million by 2050 (Administration on Aging, 2006).

The older population is likely to suffer from chronic illnesses such as arthritis, diabetes, joint disorders, and other conditions that elicit a pain response. Approximately 25%–50% of community-dwelling older adults experience persistent

TABLE 1.1   Differences Between Acute and Persistent Pain

Acute Pain	Persistent Pain
Imminent or actual tissue damage	No biological advantage
Damage to tissue limited	Functional capacity reduced
Reflex and behavioral response	Maladaptive responses common
Immobilization facilitates healing	Comorbidities such as depression, anxiety, sleep disturbances

pain (American Geriatric Society (AGS), 2002; Blyth, March, Barnabic, Jorm, Williamson, & Cousins, 2001; Mantyselka, Kumpusalo, Ahonen, Kumpusalo, Kauhanen, et al., 2001). Given the chronic and frail state of residents in long-term care facilities, it is not surprising that persistent pain occurs in 45%–80% of these residents (AGS, 2002; Ferrell, 1995). These statistics emphasize the need for understanding how pain manifests itself in older adults.

The American Geriatric Society has recognized this need and has developed guidelines related to persistent pain in older persons (AGS, 2002). Persistent pain is unfortunately under-treated in the older population for a wide variety of reasons. Consequences of untreated persistent pain include depression, anxiety, social isolation, impaired sleep, and impaired mobility. Untreated pain can lead to widespread consequences in the elderly, increasing health care utilization and costs (Ferrell, 1991). Muscle deconditioning, abnormalities in gait, falls, slow recovery, cognitive impairments, and malnutrition either contribute to or become worse with pain. Health care providers need to understand the comprehensive nature of pain in older adults (Gloth, 2001). This chapter begins this process of understanding pain in older adults by discussing the physiological mechanisms of pain in the elderly.

AGE-RELATED CHANGES IN PERCEPTION OF PAIN

Older persons often have more than one source of pain. Given the multiple causes of pain, it is often difficult to localize or target the pain source. The high prevalence of dementia, sensory impairments, compounds the problem. There is no consensus on whether perception and sensitivity of pain change with aging (Gibson & Helme, 2001). The American Geriatric Society panel concluded that no age-related changes are clinically significant in terms of perception of pain (AGS, 2002). There is a lack of studies however, in older adults, especially over age 75, examining sensitivities to pain and pain treatments. Some evidence supports the theory that good coping strategies in older adults lead to less psychological distress associated with pain (AGS, 2002). One animal study suggests that age-related changes in perception of nociceptive pain are curvilinear, and age does needs to be considered in treating pain (Finkel, Besch, Hergen, Kakarenka, Pohida, et al., 2006). Another animal study speculates that neuroimmune responses at the site of injury are developmentally regulated and less likely to produce persistent pain when injury occurs at a young age (Ririe & Eisenach, 2006).

There are multiple variables that contribute to the perception of pain in the elderly, making it difficult to determine what influences are most important. One small study examined acute and persistent pain in older adults and the influence of cognition on pain perception (Schuler, Njoo, Hetseramann, Osler, & Hauer, 2004). They found that perception of pain was independent of cognition, although cognitive impairment affected the ability to localize pain. Older individuals with chronic pain tend to use more pain descriptors, use more analgesics, and have more disability than older patients with acute pain (Schuler et al., 2004). Physiological adaptation to persistent pain is compromised because other coexisting health conditions decrease resiliency and function-ability (Ebener, 1999). Those with persistent pain often have more difficulty falling asleep and exhibit more depression and anxiety.

PHYSIOLOGY OF PAIN

The physiology of pain pathways has been widely studied, and ongoing clinical and laboratory studies continue to expand our knowledge of pain. One of the most cited theories of pain was proposed by Melzack and Wall in 1965 and is widely known as the Gate Control Theory of Pain. Their original hypothesis and framework proposed that T cells (now known as wide dynamic range neurons) carry impulses to cortical centers. These wide dynamic range neurons (WDR) could be excited by large-diameter fibers and inhibited by interneurons in the dorsal horn of the spinal cord. Although the theory explains some of the mechanisms associated with the pain process, it does not explain all of them. Pain is a complex process that involves memory, expectations, and emotions (Ferrell, 1991). Although the biopsychosocial model of pain is widely accepted, Goldberg (2007) proposes that the old nociceptive or Cartesian concept of persistent pain developed during the eighteenth century be reexamined.

The following discussion will review the general physiology of pain transmission. The reader is referred to physiology textbooks if a more in-depth and detailed physiological analysis of pain transmission is desired. At the present time there is not sufficient evidence that demonstrates that pain transmission changes significantly with aging. The main physiological change related to aging that has been documented is that A-delta fiber function decreases with aging. C fiber function remains stable, although there is some belief that older adults preferentially rely on C-fiber input.

Terms

There are several terms that need to be defined when discussing pain physiology. These terms are used frequently when describing mechanisms of pain pathways and may be helpful to review. A summary of these terms is listed in Table 1.2. Nociception and pain are often used interchangeably, but their distinction should be noted. Nociception is the reception of input into the central nervous system by sensory receptors known as nociceptors. Nociceptors provide information about injury to tissues. Not all information delivered through this system will be perceived as painful. Pain is the perception of an adverse sensation arising from a specific area of the body. It is the cognitive and subjective nature of pain that makes it difficult to manage clinically.

There are three main types of afferent nerves that are involved in pain transmission based on structure, degree of myelination, and function. *A-beta fibers* transmit sensory information regarding touch, vibration, and hair deflection. These fibers are large-diameter fibers that are myelinated, meaning that transmission along these nerves is rapid. *A-delta fibers* respond to noxious mechanical stimulation. These fibers are small-diametered, myelinated fibers and have slower conduction velocity compared to the A-beta fibers. *C polymodal nociceptors* originate at deep receptors such as ligaments, muscles, and connective tissues. These fibers are the smallest and slowest of the fibers and require greater stimulation to transmit pain impulses.

There are two major types of pain sensations, nociceptive pain and neuropathic pain. Nociceptive pain occurs from activation of free nerve endings in the skin or deeper tissues. These pain receptors, known as nociceptors, are activated by mechanical, thermal, or chemical stimuli. Nociceptive pain can be somatic or visceral in nature. Neuropathic pain arises from abnormal function of the nervous system. Partial or complete damage to nerve fibers can produce subtle abnormalities such as altered temperature or unpleasant sensation. The physiology of these two pain mechanisms will be discussed separately.

Neuropathic Pain

Neuropathic pain is very common in older adults (Ahmad & Goucke, 2002). There are many causes of neuropathic pain, often related to degeneration or

TABLE 1.2   Pain-Related Terms

Term	Definition	Comments
Nociceptive Pain	Stimulation of pain receptors (nociceptors) from visceral or somatic areas. Often described as a sharp, lancinating pain.	Arises from inflammation, mechanical deformation or ongoing injury. Responds well to analgesics and nonpharmacologic strategies.
Nociceptor	Pain receptor that is stimulated by an injury.	
Neuropathic Pain	Involves the peripheral or central nervous system. Often described as a burning, aching type pain.	Not relieved by common analgesics, but neuroleptic and antidepressant medications are often helpful.
Allodynia	Painful response to nonpainful stimuli. Activated by sensitized mechanoreceptors.	Light touch or clothing can trigger this response.
Hyperalgesia	Increased response to painful stimuli. Activated by sensitized polymodal nociceptors.	Appears to an observer as an overreaction to a painful stimulus.
Neuroplasticity	Organizational changes that develop in the brain as a result of experience.	Some experts contribute the concept of neuroplasticity to perception of neuropathic pain.
Interneuron	Neuron that communicates only with other neurons.	Interneurons are defined in terms of activity in peripheral and central nervous system.
Afferent nerve	Nerve that carries impulses toward the central nervous system.	Pain is transmitted to the dorsal horn of the spinal cord via afferent nerves.
Efferent nerve	Nerve that transmits impulses from the central nervous system toward the peripheral nervous system.	A motor neuron is an example of an efferent nerve.
Axon	Extension of a nerve cell that transmits impulses away from the cell body and branches as it terminates.	Axons synapse at its termination.
Lamina	Refers to a thin layer in the dorsal horn of the spinal column.	First order neurons terminate in the lamina I–X of the dorsal horn.

TABLE 1.3   Common Neuropathic Pain Syndromes in Older Adults

Central post-stroke

Diabetic neuropathy

Postherpetic neuralgia

Phantom limb pain

Intracostal neuralgia following thoracotomy

Ilio-inguinal neuralgia following hernia repair

Radicular spine pain

Trigeminal neuralgia

age-related changes. Table 1.3 provides examples of neuropathic conditions found in older adults. The list is not inclusive. The physiology underlying neuropathic pain involves injury to the nerve that results initially in damage or death of the axon but then develops axonal sprouting forming a neuroma (Yaksh, 2005). Neuromas are believed to cause spontaneous afferent activity. Injury to the nerve can cause increased dorsal horn excitability, altered inhibitory control, and reorganization of nonneuronal cells. An individual suffering from neuropathic pain may experience hyperalgesia or allodynia. Hyperalgesia is increased pain sensation, whereas allodynia is pain sensation with nonnoxious stimuli. The four most common types of neuropathic pain are direct stimulation of pain-sensitive neurons, automatic firing of damaged nerves, deafferentation, and sympathetically mediated pain (Belgrade, 1999).

Direct Stimulation of Pain-Sensitive Neurons

Neuropathic pain can be caused by direct stimulation of C-nociceptors. Stimulation can be in response to mechanical stretching, compression, or chemical mediators. A tumor or mass compressing a nerve complex or spinal cord will be perceived in the area of nerve distribution for those fibers. Release of chemical mediators secondary to the inflammatory response in disc herniation, for example, can irritate adjacent nerve roots.

Automatic Firing of Damaged Nerves

Nerves that are damaged due to disease or injury can result in spontaneous impulse firing from the site of injury or along the damaged nerve. This type of nerve pain is seen in patients with large-fiber diabetic neuropathy, chemotherapy, pesticides, or any type of unrelenting neuropathic pain. Neuropathic pain resulting from automatic firing of damaged nerves can be described as lancinating, stabbing, or shooting pain. When multiple nerve fibers are affected and fire asynchronously, the pain will be described as a continuous burning-type pain (Belgrade, 1999).

Deafferentation

Pain transmission follows an upward route from the area of injury or damage to the spinal cord, brain stem, and cortex, relaying the impulse from level-ordered neurons. Interruption at any level of the ordered neurons can result in irritability and aberrant firing of nerves. Examples of this type of neuropathic pain include phantom limb pain, diabetic neuropathy, post-herpetic neuropathy, or peripheral nerve trauma. Central post-stroke syndrome is an example of ongoing neuropathic pain that is experienced at one site but is generated at the infarct site further along the pain transmission route.

Sympathetic Mediated Pain

Sympathetic mediated pain refers to autonomic nervous system activity that occurs with pain stimulation. Sympathetic response may be triggered initially by the inflammatory response. The sympathetic activity can continue in a regional versus a dermatomal response area. The sympathetic nerves release norepinepherine, which can further stimulate C polymodal nociceptors and subsequently further stimulate sympathetic mediated pain. The person experiences diaphoresis, skin temperature changes, and altered peripheral circulation along with persistent neuropathic pain. As the sympathetic cycle persists, chronic regional pain syndrome (CRPS), previously known as reflex sympathetic dystrophy (RSD), can develop.

Other Mechanisms

Neuropathic pain involves changes in the peripheral and central nervous systems (Charlton, 2005). There is some evidence that changes in the sodium channels within the peripheral nervous system promote the ectopic activity pain transmission (Waxman, 1999). Blocking of these sodium channels with the use of local anesthetics and anticonvulsant medications has shown effectiveness in reducing neuropathic pain. Sodium channels have also been found in C-fibers, which holds potential for future pharmacologic intervention. Other observations and potential explanations for neuropathic pain include presence of nerve growth factor that may influence responsiveness and regrowth of sensory neurons during inflammation and nerve injury (Charlton, 2005).

Central nervous system involvement in neuropathic pain centers on the concept of neuroplasticity. Neuroplasticity refers to organizational changes in the brain in response to experience. Injury to the nerve and injury-related areas undergo long-term neuroplastic changes, enhancing pain sensation such as hyperalgesia or allodynia (Zhou, 2007). The anterior cingulate cortex (ACC) in the forebrain is believed to be a major area for pain-related perception, in that it may serve as a key area for pain interacting with other cognitive functions. The ACC contains many pyramidal cells, interneurons, and nonpyramidal cells. Pyramidal cells exhibit excitatory activity whereas nonpyramidal cells are inhibitory neurons containing gamma aminobutyric acid. The pyramidal cells project to the periaqueductal gray and hypothalamus and may contribute to descending modulation (Zhou, 2007). Pain modulation and the role of neurotransmitters will be discussed later in this chapter.

Nociceptive Pain

Nociceptors located in somatic tissues are dense and can easily localize pain. For example, when someone cuts their finger, the person is fully aware of where the laceration occurred. Nociceptors located in visceral organs are less dense, and pain experienced from these areas is more diffuse or referred. There are several causes of visceral pain including ischemia, chemical damage, spasm, distention, or stretching of connective tissue (Table 1.4). When visceral pain is referred to the body's surface, the individual localizes the pain in the dermatomal segment from embryonic development, not where the organ is currently located. A classic example is left shoulder pain with laceration of the spleen.

Impulses from nociceptors located in free nerve endings are transmitted to the dorsal horn of the spinal cord via myelinated fibers (A-delta) or

TABLE 1.4   Causes of Visceral Pain

Cause	Example
Ischemia of visceral tissue	Chest pain
Chemical damage to viscera	Peritonitis
Spasm of smooth muscle	Intestinal spasms
Visceral distention	Distended bladder
Stretching of connective tissue	Abdominal pain

slower unmyelinated fibers known as C polymodal nociceptors. The A-delta fibers appear responsible for sending signals to the brain that interpret pain as sharp and lancinating. The slower C fibers transmit the secondary pain sensation, that of a burning, aching type pain that persists after the initial injury (Serpell, 2005). These enter the spinal cord via the dorsal horn and synapse in lamina I, V, and X. The wide dynamic range neurons (WDR) in lamina V are thought to be "sensory-discriminative" and project into the ventrobasal thalamus, where another synapse occurs before projecting to the somata-sensory cortex (Yaksh, 2005). Marginal, nociceptive specific neurons ascend from lamina I in the dorsal horn and project contralaterally to ventrobasal and medial thalamus. Input from these neurons appears to have a role in the "affective-motivational" component of the pain pathway (Yaksh, 2005).

There are three major ascending pathways that transmit nociceptive information, the spinothalamic, spinoreticular, and spinomesocephalic tracts. The *spinothalamic* tract is the main nociceptive tract that originates from neurons found in laminae I–VII and X and ascend contralaterally to the ventral thalamus. The neuron entering the dorsal horn is referred to as the first ordered neuron. The neuron projecting to the thalamus is known as the second order neuron, and the neuron projecting to the somatosensory cortex is the third order neuron. Table 1.5 identifies the ordered neurons and their projections. Interneuron activity and neurotransmitter release occurs at these synapses. The *spinoreticular* tract is made up of axons from laminae VII and VIII. Some axons cross the midline, while others project upward uncrossed. These axons terminate in both the reticular formation and the thalamus. Neurons in laminae I, VI–VIII, and X ascend contralaterally in the *spinomesencephalic* tract to the mesencephalic reticular formation, the lateral periaqueductal gray and some areas in the midbrain. Other ascending transmission pathways include the *dorsal column post-synaptic spinomedullar tract* and the *propriospinal multisynaptic ascending system*. Pain transmission via multiple tracts provides support for use of multiple therapies in managing pain. Many C fibers terminate in reticular areas of brain-stem and intralaminar nuclei of the thalamus. These

TABLE 1.5   Afferent Pain Transmission

Neuron	Synapse
First order neuron	Dorsal horn of spinal cord
Second order neuron	Thalamus
Third order neuron	Somatosensory cortex

areas have a strong arousal effect on the nervous system and may help explain why patients have sleep disturbances with severe pain.

Neurotransmitters

The nociceptive signals from the dorsal horn neurons are transmitted by chemical means. Several amino acids and peptides have been identified as excitatory or inhibitory neurotransmitters. Table 1.6 identifies some of the afferent neurotransmitters. Some peptides that have been identified include cholecystokinin, dynorphin, somatostain, bombesin, vasoactive intestinal peptides, and substance P. Glutamate, an amino acid, has a role in excitation. Glutamate is most likely the neurotransmitter associated with A-delta pain, and substance P with C fiber pain (Guyton & Hall, 2006). Other excitatory neurotransmitters include bradykinin, serotonin, histamine, potassium ions, acids, ACTH, and proteolytic enzymes. Prostaglandins and substance P enhance the sensitivity of pain endings but do not directly excite them (Guyton & Hall, 2006). The nonadapting nature of pain receptors leads to hypersensitivity.

Interneurons, neurons that communicate only with other neurons, play an important role in releasing excitatory or inhibitory neurotransmitters (Chao & Hart, 2003). There are actually two different definitions for interneurons, depending on whether one is referring to the peripheral or central nervous system. In the peripheral nervous system, an interneuron refers exclusively to neurons that only communicate to other neurons and have no central pathways or processes. These interneurons signal release of excitatory or inhibitory neurotransmitters pre- or post-synaptically. In the central nervous system, interneurons can also refer to a group of locally projecting neurons that release neurotransmitters. One group of locally projecting neurons releases the inhibitory neurotransmitter gamma aminobutyric acid and plays a role in pain modulation.

TABLE 1.6   **Examples of Afferent Neurotransmitters**

Neurotransmitter	Type
Substance P	Peptide
Adenosine triphosphate (ATP)	Purine
Aspartate	Excitatory amino acid
Glutamate	Excitatory amino acid

Pain Modulation

Pain transmission not only involves ascending nerve transmission but also descending pathways that allow the individual to react to the pain sensation. These descending pathways can be manipulated or enhanced to modulate the pain response. For example, stimulation of A-beta fibers from peripheral tactile receptors can depress pain transmission. Examples of this type of modulation include rubbing a painful area, applying liniment ointments, or use of acupuncture.

These descending pathways were discovered by stimulating areas in the brain, particularly the paraventricular gray area and ventrobasal area of thalamus. It was found that stimulation of these areas inhibited the nociceptive neurons in the dorsal horn of the spinal column.

The main descending modulating pathway in the midbrain has three basic components. First, there are neurons in the midbrain, in particular the periventricular and periaqueductal gray matter that have excitatory connections in the medulla that is serotonergic. This excitation releases serotonin, a neurotransmitter with inhibitory properties. Second, neurons in the medulla make inhibitory connections in the dorsal horn, particularly laminae I, II, and V, where the afferent nociceptors terminate. These connections include spinothalamic tract neurons that respond to painful stimuli. The third component involves local circuits in the dorsal horn that mediate the modulatory actions of the descending pathways.

A second major descending pathway occurs in the pons and involves norepinepherine. The descending pathways from the midbrain and pons are crucial links in the supraspinal modulation of nociceptive transmission. The descending serotonergic and noradrenergic axons contact the dendrites of the spinothalamic tract.

Another central mechanism of pain modulation involves endogenous opioid peptides. These peptides play a role in modulating nociceptive transmission at the level of the primary afferent synapse in the dorsal horn. Many peptides have been identified as endogenous opiates and fall within three classes: enkephalins, beta endorphins, and dynorphins. The superficial dorsal horn has a high density of enkephalin and dynorphin interneurons close to the terminals of nociceptive afferents and dendrites. The opiate peptides bind to specific membrane receptors. Three major classes of opiate receptors, mu, kappa, and delta, have been identified. The beta endorphins are active at mu receptors, whereas enkephains are active at mu and delta receptors and dynorphin endogenous opiates are active at kappa receptors. Mu receptors are more prevalent at the terminals of nociceptive afferents and dendrites of post-synaptic neurons. The mu receptors inhibit the excitatory neurotransmitter glutamate. Morphine is a potent agonist of mu receptors. Morphine inhibits interneuron that releases gamma aminobutyric acid (GABA). Descending inhibition of the spinothalamic tract is mediated by activation of the enkephalin interneurons in the dorsal horn. Discovery of these endogenous opioids led to the development of epidural and intrathecal delivery systems. Modulation of nociceptive transmission at the level of the primary afferent occurs with the combination of pre-synaptic and post-synaptic actions.

SUMMARY

Pain is a common concern of older adults. Pain can be acute or persistent. Physiological adaptation to persistent pain is compromised because exacerbations of other coexisting health conditions decrease resiliency and functionability (Ebener, 1999). Persistent pain can result in deconditioning, sleep disturbances, and poor nutrition. Understanding the physiological mechanisms of pain transmission and modulation helps the health care professional to develop an appropriate pain management plan.

REFERENCES

Administration on Aging. (2004). Aging into the 21st century. Retrieved December 26, 2007, from www.aos.gov/prof/Statistics/future_growth/aging21/demography.asp.

Ahmad, M., & Goucke, C. R. (2002). Management strategies for the treatment of neuropathic pain in the elderly. *Drugs and Aging, 19*(12), 930–945.

American Geriatric Society. (AGS). (2002). The management of persistent pain in older persons. AGS Panel on Persistent Pain in Older Persons. *Journal of the American Geriatic Society, 50,* S205–S224.

Belgrade, M. J. (1999). Following the clues to neuropathic pain. Distribution and other leads reveal the cause and the treatment approach. *Postgraduate Medical Journal, 106*(6). Retrieved December 26, 2007, from www.postgradmed.com/issues/1999/11_99/neuropathic.htm.

Blyth, F. M., March, L. M, Barnabic A. J., Jorm, L. R., Williamson, M., & Cousins, M. J. (2001). Chronic pain in Australia: A prevalence study. *Pain, 89,* 127–134.

Chao, M. Y., & Hart, A. C. (2003). Sensory biology: How the nose knows. *Current Biology, 13*(6), R226–R228.

Charlton, J. E. (2005). *Core curriculum for professional education in pain.* Seattle: IASP Press.

Ebener, M. K. (1999). Older adults living with chronic pain: an opportunity for improvement. *Journal of Nursing Care and Quality, 13*(4), 1–7.

Federal Interagency Forum on Age-Related Statistics. (2004). *Older Americans 2004: Key indicators of well being.* Washington, DC: U.S. Government Printing Office.

Ferrell, B. A. (1991). Pain management in elderly people. *Journal of the American Geriatric Society, 39,* 64–73.

Ferrell, B. A. (1995). Pain evaluation and management in the nursing home. *Annals of Internal Medicine, 23,* 681–687.

Finkel, J. C., Besch, V. G., Hergen, A., Kakarenka, J., Pohida, T., Melzer, J. M., et al. (2006). Effects of aging on current vocalization threshold in mice measured by a novel Nociception assay. *Anesthesiology, 105*(2), 360–369.

Gibson, S. J., & Helme, R. D. (2001). Age-related differences in pain perception and report. *Clinical Geriatric Medicine, 17,* 433–456.

Gloth, F. M. (2001). Pain management in older adults; prevention and treatment. *Journal of the American Geriatric Society, 49,* 188–199.

Goldberg, J. S. (2007). Revisiting the Cartesian model of pain. *Medical Hypotheses, 9.* doi:10.1016/j.mehy.2007.08.014.

Guyton, A. C., & Hall, J. E. (2006). *Textbook of medical physiology* (11th ed., pp. 598–609). Philadelphia: Elsevier.

Mantyselka, P., Kumpusalo, E., Ahonen, R., Kumpusalo, A., Kauhanen, J., Viinamaki, H., et al. (2001). Pain as a reason to visit the doctor: A study in Finnish primary health care. *Pain, 89,* 175–180.

Melzack, R., & Wall, P. D. (1965). Pain mechanisms: A new theory. *Science, 150,* 971–979.

Ririe, D. G., & Eisenach, J. C. (2006). Age-dependent responses to nerve injury-induced mechanical allodynia. *Anesthesiology, 104*(2), 344–350.

Schuler, M., Njoo, N., Hestermann, M., Osler, P., & Hauer, K. (2004). Acute and chronic pain in geriatrics: Clinical characteristics of pain and the influence of cognition *American Academy of Pain Medicine, 5*(3), 253–259.

Serpell, M. (2005). Anatomy, physiology and pharmacology of pain. *Anaesthesia and Intensive Care Medicine, 6,* 7–10.

Waxman, S. (1999). The molecular pathophysiology of pain: Abnormal expression of sodium channel genes and its contribution to hyperexcitability of primary sensory neurons. *Pain, 6,* S133–S140.

Yaksh, T. L. (2005). Physiology and pharmacology of post tissue injury processing. Madison, WI: Comprehensive Pain Board Review.

Zhou, M. (2007). Neuronal mechanism for neuropathic pain. *Molecular pain, 3.* Retrieved December 26, 2007, from www.molecularpain.com/content/3/1/14.

CHAPTER 2

Common Pain Syndromes in Older Adults

Michaelene P. Jansen

There are many causes of pain in older persons. Some causes are the result of physiological aspects of aging and some result from disease or pathological conditions (Weiner, 2007). This chapter will focus on common pain syndromes that occur in older adults. For the most part, these common pain syndromes are persistent pain syndromes, although there are also many chronic conditions that can cause acute pain, such as a compression fracture resulting from osteoporosis. The most common cause of persistent, nonmalignant pain in older adults is related to the musculoskeletal system, including arthritis and myofascial pain syndromes (Podichetty, Mazanec, & Biscup, 2003). This chapter will examine several pain syndromes common in older adults. The syndromes described in this chapter are not exhaustive but represent a sample of painful conditions commonly seen in the elderly. A brief description of each condition or syndrome will be presented with a general management plan for each condition. Details of treatment modalities are presented in subsequent chapters.

It is important for the health care professional to recognize origins of pain in older adults. Accurately identifying the condition or syndrome causing the pain is crucial to identifying the pain generators to determine an appropriate management plan. Specific assessment questions and follow-up can reduce or shorten the length of pain. It is important to treat ongoing, persistent pain to maintain quality of life and mobility. Early recognition and treatment is critical to avoid undesired consequences of persistent pain such as depression, disrupted sleep, limited function, anxiety, and dysfunctional relationships. The overall goal is to increase functional ability and reduce pain severity.

MUSCULOSKELETAL PAIN

Studies have shown that the prevalence and intensity of musculoskeletal pain increases with age (Riley, Wade, Robinson, & Price, 2000). However, there are conflicting reports as to intensity of pain changes with aging. Pain associated with musculoskeletal disorders and limited mobility affect function and quality of life in older adults (Staud, 2007). Improving mobility and function by reducing musculoskeletal pain is a goal in treatment. Musculoskeletal causes of pain are fairly well known and understood by the general population and health care providers. Some of the more common musculoskeletal disorders prevalent in older adults will be discussed briefly in this section.

Osteoarthritis

Osteoarthritis is the most common musculoskeletal condition in the older adult. It is estimated that 40% of patients over the age of 80 have symptomatic arthritis (Harrington & Schneider, 2006). Osteoarthritis is characterized by the breakdown of joint cartilage. Cartilage cushions ends of bones, allowing for easy and pain-free movement of joints. As the cartilage loses its elasticity, it becomes more damaged and prone to injury. As the cartilage wears, the underlying bone thickens and bony spurs or growths can develop. Bone pieces or chips can break away from the bone and float into the joint space. As the cartilage breaks down, the synovioum becomes inflamed. As the inflammatory process ensues, chemical mediators such as cytokines are released and cause further breakdown of the cartilage.

Several factors can contribute to the development of osteoarthritis. These include age, excess weight, joint injury, and joint stress. As one ages, the cartilage loses its elasticity and provides less cushion for the bones. Excessive weight can put undue stress on the cartilage and bone. Prior injury or joint stress from over-activity, strenuous physical work, or sports has contributed to osteoarthritis.

Maintaining activity and joint mobility have benefit in maintaining quality of life and reducing pain. However, pain associated with activity, particularly physical activity, limits or restricts the intent or effort. Knee buckling is very common in osteoarthritis of the knee and is associated with weak quadriceps muscles (Felson, Niu, McClennan, Sack, Aliabadi, et al., 2007). There is an increased effort to develop exercise programs that increase mobility and muscle strength and promote balance and gait in older adults. Water exercises and warm water therapy reduce the stress on joints. Unfortunately, not all older adults have access to pools or water therapy programs.

As the cartilage deteriorates and the disease progresses, pain persists. Current treatment for osteoarthritis includes exercise, weight control, balance of activity and rest, nonpharmacological and pharmacologic treatment of pain, complementary and alternative therapies, and surgery.

Pharmacologic agents that have been used in the treatment of osteoarthritis include nonsteroidal anti-inflammatory drugs such as naproxen and ibuprofen. A study comparing refecoxib, celecoxib, acetaminophen, and nabumetone demonstrated efficacy within six days of therapy and lasting for six weeks (Battisti, Katz, Weaver, Matsumoto, Kivitz, et al., 2004). This study was conducted prior to the recall of refecoxib. The long-term use of these medications in older adults, particularly if they are on anticoagulants or aspirin therapy, needs further study. Selective COX-2 inhibitors such as celecoxib also need to be used with caution, particularly if the older adult has cardiovascular disease. Lidocaine patches have shown to improve outcomes for low back pain and osteoarthritis when compared to selective COX-2 inhibitors and traditional NSAID therapy (Galer, Oleka, & Gammaitoni, 2005). Tramadol and opioid analgesics may be indicated for severe arthritic pain. Extended release forms of mild opiate analgesics provide ongoing therapeutic drug levels. As always, caution is needed when using opiates in older adults due to adverse drug effects and drug interactions.

As osteoarthritis progresses, radiographic imaging of joints will detect changes in joint space fairly late in the disease. There is some evidence that changes in the biochemical structure of cartilage may be able to be detected through magnetic resonance imaging. Early detection of the disease, along with the development of disease-modifying drugs for osteoarthritis, as well as improved cartilage resurfacing techniques hold promise for the early treatment of osteoarthritis.

Surgical interventions for joint replacement have made technological advances in recent years. Minimally invasive joint replacements have improved postoperative recovery and pain in older adults.

Spondylosis/Spinal Stenosis

Spinal osteoarthritis is called spondylosis and can affect the cervical, thoracic, and lumbar spine. Spondylosis occurs in 6% of the population. Bone spurs can develop, causing narrowing of the spinal canal, which causes *spinal stenosis*. As the spinal canal narrows, the spinal cord or its nerves can become compressed and may require decompression surgery. Minimally invasive decompression surgery for lumbar spinal stenosis has decreased hospital stays, decreased use of opiate analgesics, and reduced readmission rates (Podichetty, Spears, Isaacs, Booher, & Buscup, 2006). Conservative measures include pharmacologic treatment or epidural spinal injection. Spinal interventions are discussed in detail in Chapter 10.

Spondylothesis is a degenerative process in which a vertebrae slips forward onto the next vertebrae. Mild cases of spondylothesis can be managed conservatively. More severe cases may require spinal fusion.

Degenerative Disc Disease

The intervertebral disc undergoes biochemical and degenerative changes with aging. The degeneration of spinal discs, particularly in the lumbar spine, is a common cause of low back pain that increases with aging. It is hypothesized that the substance proteoglycans decreases significantly and is a major factor in intervertebral disc degeneration (Podichetty, 2007). In addition to the decrease in proteoglycans, numerous inflammatory mediators play a role in the degradation of articular cartilage. These biochemical changes lead to structural vertebral damage and loss of normal vertebral function.

Vertebral Compression Fractures

Vertebral compression fractures occur in 25% of all postmenopausal women and increases to 40% in women over 80 (Old & Calvert, 2004). Older men also suffer from vertebral compression fractures, but at a much lower rate of incidence. The main contributing factor to compression fractures is osteoporosis. Clinical manifestations include sudden onset of localized pain that improves with rest and increases with any movement or activity.

Not all vertebral compression fractures are diagnosed. Only about a third of the fractures are documented. Most individuals attribute their pain to arthritis. The most common areas for compression fractures to occur are between T8-T12 and L1-L4. Often the compression fractures occur at multiple levels. Computerized tomography and magnetic resonance imaging, along with a bone scan, are used to help diagnose compression fractures.

Treatment for stable fractures is conservative therapy consisting of short-term bedrest, analgesics for pain control, and close monitoring of bowel function. A common complication of a vertebral compression fracture is constipation and bowel obstruction. Calcitonin-salmon (Miacalcin) nasal spray, muscle relaxants, back braces, and physical therapy may also be helpful.

Percutaneous vertebroplasty may be beneficial for patients not responding to conservative therapy. Acrylic cement is injected into the compressed vertebrae to strengthen and stabilize the fracture. If successful, the pain is decreased immediately. Vertebroplasty does not restore the height of the vertebrae but kyphoplasty, where cement is placed into the cavity using a high-pressure balloon, will restore vertebral height. Kyphoplasty is currently undergoing evaluation and is not widely available.

It goes without saying that the best treatment for vertebral compression fracture is prevention of osteoporosis. Increasing bone mineral density at an early age with healthy lifestyles will reduce the incidence of osteoporosis and vertebral compression fractures.

Myofascial Pain

Myofascia is the thin translucent film that wraps around muscles tissue. It supports the musculature and gives shape to the body. There are three layers of myofascia, superficial, deep, and subserous (Bennett, 2007). The myofascia can become a taut band in a muscle or in multiple muscles. This taut band is known as a trigger point. Trigger points can be palpated and feel like tight knots. These trigger points can be quite painful. Latent trigger points elicit pain when they are manipulated or aroused. Active trigger points are painful without being palpated or manipulated. The pain can be localized or referred pain.

Myofascial pain can be persistent and can be aggravated by poor posture, poor body mechanics, repetitive work or exercise, or anything that decreases oxygen to the muscle. In the past, myofascial pain was recognized as a syndrome meaning that a certain set of signs and symptoms occur together. However, recently, chronic myofascial pain has been recognized as a disease, and causes of myofascial pain has been identified.

As with any chronic pain condition, various events or stimuli can trigger myofascial pain. In general, any event that puts stress on the muscle can result in a trigger point. Some more common triggers include impaired sleep, gum chewing, cigarette smoking, dental work, exposure to chemicals or heavy metals, inhalant or food allergies, nutritional deficiencies, malabsorption, chronic infection, alcohol ingestion, and stress.

Myofascial pain can occur in all age groups. Statistics are not currently available to determine its prevalence in the older population, other than that it is a common problem. Descriptions of myofascial pain include muscle tightness, tenderness, stiffness, limitation of movement, "knotty" muscles, limited range of motion, and local twitch. Trigger points can be easily identified by palpation. Gentle massage can relieve the discomfort at times but can also activate latent trigger points, causing pain.

Since myofascial pain can be localized or referred, it is helpful to have a good working knowledge of muscle and nerve distribution. For example, if an individual has low back pain due to a degenerative L4-L5 disc, it would not be unusual to palpate a trigger band in the paraspinous muscles on the affected side. The same would hold true if an older person had degenerative changes of the cervical spine. The person would feel tightness or discomfort in the shoulder area on the affected side. This area would correlate with the supraspinous or the trapezius muscles.

Several books and self-help guides are available to help not only the clinician, but also the individual to treat the myofascial pain (Davies, Davies, & Simmons, 2004; Finando & Finando, 2005; Starlanyl & Copeland, 2001). Treatment options for myofascial pain include myofascial release, massage, heat therapy, acupuncture, and trigger point injections (Ga, Choi, Park, & Yoon, 2007; Sprenger & Tolle, 2007). Treatment for myofascial pain is discussed further in Chapter 7.

Fibromyalgia

Fibromyalgia is a persistent pain syndrome that is characterized by widespread muscle aches and pain. Muscles stiffness, fatigue, tenderness of the soft tissues, and sleep disturbances also accompany this syndrome (National Fibromyalgia Association, 2007). The American College of Rheumatology published diagnostic criteria in 1990 to facilitate the accurate diagnosis of this syndrome. Exhibit 2.1 lists the tender point sites that must be present in at least 11 of the 18 sites with approximately 4 kg force of digital palpation.

Approximately 7% of women between the ages of 60–79 have fibromyalgia compared to 3–6% of the general population (Wolfe, Ross, Anderson, Russell, & Hebert, 1995). It is important to note that myofascial pain and fibromyalgia can be used inaccurately. Chronic myofascial pain has distinct trigger points, whereas fibromyalgia has tender points. Individuals with chronic myofascial pain may also have fibromyalgia. Individuals with fibromyalgia have muscle pain and almost all report fatigue (Wolfe, Smythe, Yunas, Bennett, Bombardier, et al., 1990). Other accompanying symptoms include insomnia, joint pain, headaches, numbness and tingling, and restless legs (Endresen, 2007). It is interesting to note that according to the American College of Rheumatology, only 20% of patients have major depression associated with fibromyalgia.

EXHIBIT 2.1 TENDER POINTS IN FIBROMYALGIA

Pain in 11 of 18 Tender Point Sites on Digital Palpation

Definition: Pain, on digital palpation, must be present in at least 11 of the following 18 tender point sites:

- Occiput (2): at the suboccipital muscle insertions
- Low cervical (2): at the anterior aspects of the intertransverse spaces at C5-C7
- Trapezius (2): at the midpoint of the upper border
- Supraspinatus (2): at origins, above the scapula spine near the medial border
- Second rib (2): upper lateral to the second costochondral junction
- Lateral epicondyle (2): 2 cm distal to the epicondyles
- Gluteal (2): in upper outer quadrants of buttocks in anterior fold of muscle
- Greater trochanter (2): posterior to the trochanteric prominence
- Knee (2): at the medial fat pad proximal to the joint line

Digital palpation should be performed with an approximate force of 4 kg. A tender point has to be painful at palpation, not just "tender."

It is sometimes difficult for patients to obtain full diagnostic and treatment attention from health care providers because of the belief among some practitioners that fibromyalgia is ill-defined and a catch-all term when a diagnosis cannot be determined. Treatment options are not always effective, and due to the chronic nature of the syndrome, compliance to treatment regimens can be lacking. Therefore, caring for patients with fibromyalgia can be frustrating not only for patients and their families but also for health care providers.

There is strong evidence that low-dose tricyclic antidepressants or cyclobenzeprine given at night along with cardiovascular exercise, cognitive behavioral therapy, and patient education are beneficial to the patient. There is modest evidence that tramadol, selective serotonin reuptake inhibitors (SSRIs) such as fluoxetine, and dual reuptake inhibitors (SNRI) such as venlafaxine (Effexor®) and duloxetine (Cymbalta®), as well as some anticonvulsants such as gabapentin (Neurontin®) are useful in treating fibromyalgia. Pregabalin (Lyrica®) has recently been approved for the treatment of fibromyalgia. There is also modest evidence that strength training, acupuncture, hypnotherapy, biofeedback, and balneotherapy can be useful as well. There is no evidence for the use of opioids, corticosteroids, nonsteroidal anti-inflammatory drugs, thyroid hormone, melatonin, trigger point injections, or flexibility exercise (Goldenberg, Burckhart, & Crofford, 2004; American Pain Society, 2005).

NEUROPATHIC PAIN SYNDROMES

Radicular Pain

Radicular pain caused by disc disease either at the cervical or lumbar level is the most common cause of neuropathic pain in persons over 30 (Khoromi, Patsalides, Parada, Salehi, Meegan, et al., 2005). Degenerative changes in the spine can impinge on nerve roots causing a radicular component of the pain. Radicular pain transmits an aching, burning type pain along the nerve and dermatomal distribution. The term radiculitis refers to pain radiating from the nerve root. Radiculopathy refers to neurological deficits that occur with damage to the spinal nerve. Radiculopathy is seen clinically by decreased deep tendon reflexes or extremity weakness.

Treatment of radicular pain can be conservative or, if radiculopathy is present, surgical intervention may be warranted. Pharmacologic treatment includes neuropathic medications such as gabapentin or pregabalin. Epidural steroid injections may be beneficial. Persistent lumbar radiculitis may respond to spinal cord stimulation.

Peripheral Neuropathy

Peripheral neuropathy is aching, burning-type pain that occurs in the peripheral nervous system. In the older population, the most common types of peripheral neuropathy occur from peripheral vascular disease, diabetic neuropathy, and post-herpetic neuralgia. There are other causes of peripheral neuropathy such as post-thoracotomy pain, post-radiation pain, phantom limb pain, trigeminal neuralgia, central post-stroke, and nerve compression or entrapment.

Diabetic Peripheral Neuropathy (DPN)

Diabetes is the leading cause of neuropathy in the United States. Type 2 diabetes is under-diagnosed and often occurs after micro- or macrovascular complications are well advanced. Peripheral neuropathy is present in fifty percent of diabetics. The primary risk factor for diabetic neuropathy is hyperglycemia. Therefore glycemic control of diabetes is essential in decreasing the risk of diabetic neuropathy. Four types of diabetic neuropathy have been identified, including peripheral, autonomic, proximal, and focal neuropathy. Although pain can occur with all forms of diabetic neuropathy, this section will focus on diabetic peripheral neuropathy.

Diabetic peripheral neuropathy (DPN) affects large and small afferent nerve fibers and is insidious in its progression. DPN begins in the distal extremities as a painless loss or change in sensation. Typical symptoms include numbness, tingling, and a burning sensation. However, sharp pain, hypersensitivity to pain, and loss of balance and coordination can occur with diabetic peripheral neuropathy. As the disease progresses, the pain becomes refractory and excruciating as a result of nerve ischemia, dysfunction, and death (Duby, Campbell, Setter, White, & Rasmussen, 2004).

The optimal treatment for diabetic peripheral neuropathy is prevention. The United Kingdom Prospective Diabetic Study (UKPDS) and the Diabetes Clinical Control Trial (DCCT) clearly demonstrated the importance of glycemic control in the prevention of diabetic complications. Since the progression of DPN is insidious, the American Diabetic Association provides, as one standard of practice, annual screening for DPN using pinprick sensation, temperature, vibration perception, and 10-g monofilament pressure sensation at the distal plantar aspect of both great toes (American Diabetes Association, 2007). Optimal glycemic control is also an important preventative factor.

Pharmacologic treatment for DPN targets symptom management rather than modifying the underlying disease. Table 2.1 summarizes the most common medications used in treating persistent pain associated with diabetic peripheral neuropathy. The reader is referred to Chapter 9 for a more detailed discussion of these medications. Specific attributes of the medications in relation to DPN will be highlighted in this chapter.

Anticonvulsants such as gabapentin and pregabalin have shown significant efficacy in DPN (Duby et al., 2007). Dosages of these medications may need to be adjusted in older adults. This may pose some difficulty, as one study found that pregabalin administered in normal doses (150 mg/day) did not show any difference compared to placebo, but when increased to 600 mg/day, pregabalin was effective and tolerated well (Richter, Portenoy, Sharma, Lamoreaux, Bockbrader, et al., 2005). Although the mean age in this study was 57, the implications for older adults are not clear. Tricyclic antidepressants and selective serotonin-reuptake inhibitors (SSRIs) have been trialed in the treatment of DPN. SSRIs did not demonstrate to have significant effectiveness compared to placebo. Tricyclic medications such as amitriptyline and nortriptyline reduced pain and paresthesia associated with DPN, but drug interactions and side effects limit the use with older adults. Other antidepressants such as venlafaxine have been examined with small sample sizes, and pain relief with doses between 150 and 225 mg daily have been reported (Davis & Smith, 1999). Duloxetine, a serotonin and norepinepherine uptake inhibitor has shown efficacy in treating DPN. One study demonstrated the cost-effectiveness of using

TABLE 2.1   Pharmacologic Treatment for Symptomatic DPN

Class	Examples	Dose	Comment
Anticonvulsants	Gabapentin (Neurontin®)	300–1200 mg tid	Begin titration with very low doses due to somnolence and mental blurring. May need to begin with 100 mg at night and titrate upward in older adults
	Pregabalin (Lyrica®)	100 mg tid	Begin at 50 mg tid and titrate slowly
	Carbamazepine	200–400 mg tid	Not considered a first line drug
5-hydroxytryptamine and norepinephrine uptake inhibitor	Duloxetine (Cymbalta®)	60–120 mg daily	Caution if used with other SSRI antidepressants
Tricyclic medications	Amitriptyline	10–75 mg at bedtime	Caution with older adults due to anticholinergic side effects
	Nortriptyline	25–75 mg at bedtime	
	Imipramine	25–75 mg at bedtime	
Substance P inhibitor	Capsaisin cream	0.025–0.075% 3 to 4 times daily	Burning sensation at site of application

Adapted from American Diabetic Association Standards of Medical Care in Diabetes (2007).

duloxetine compared to routine treatment of DPN (Wu, Birnbaum, Mareva, Le, Robinson, et al., 2005). NSAIDs and opioid analgesics have also been used in the treatment of DPN but have a limited role in light of other medications available.

Other medications have been trialed but have not gained wide acceptance due to the lack of efficacy or adverse effects. These medications include mexiletine, levodopa, and dextromethorphan and lamotrigine (Lamictal®) However, reports from two double-blind trials with lamotrigine did not show any alteration in nerve conduction and results were similar to placebo (Blum, Biton, & Tuchman, 2007). Lacosamide, a novel anticonvulsant, is currently in phase three clinical trials and may hold some promise in the treatment of diabetic peripheral neuropathy (Beyreuther, Freitag, Heers, Krebsfanger, Scharkenecker, et al., 2007).

Complementary and alternative therapies such as electrostimulation and percutaneous electrical nerve stimulation have been reported to help reduce the pain associated with DPN. A double-blind study using IV infusion of thioctic acid (lipoic acid) 600 mg daily demonstrated clinically significant pain relief in patients with DPN but is not practical because the half life for oral alpha lipoic acid is less than 5 minutes (Duby et al., 2004).

One of the difficulties in effectively treating patients with diabetic peripheral neuropathy is that the burden of illness is significant (Gore, Brandenburg, Hoffman, Tai, & Stacy, 2005). This study demonstrated that moderate to high levels of pain, multiple drug regimens, health resources use, and activity/work restrictions contributed to the burden of illness. Noncompliance has also been suggested as a factor in contributing to the burden of DPN.

Phantom Limb Pain

Phantom limb pain (PLP) occurs in 50%–80% of amputations (Richardson, Glenn, Horgan, & Nurmikko, 2006). Over half of limb amputations are due to diabetes. Phantom limb pain is not a new phenomenon. It was first described in 1871 and is often described as a stabbing, squeezing, cramping, shooting, burning type pain. Some patients report that fatigue, weather pattern changes, and anxiety exacerbate their pain. PLP can be intermittent or constant. Pain develops in 75% of patients within the first few days following surgery (Nikolajsen & Jensen, 2001). Most patients report a decrease in PLP by one year post-amputation, although it remains present (Ehde, Jensen, Williams, & Smith, 2007).

Several theories exist regarding the etiology of PLP. These theories include loss of peripheral nerve injury, regeneration of nerves, neuroma formation, alteration in ion channel activity at site of injury, deafferentation, neuroplasticity, or organizational changes in the brain and psychological response (Nikolajsen & Jensen, 2001). It is most likely that there are several contributing factors to PLP rather than just one factor. Spinal plasticity and cerebral reorganization are two mechanisms receiving more attention lately.

There is some speculation that age is related to a decreased perception of phantom limb pain, suggesting that pain intensity and function diminish with age. Molton and colleagues (2007) found that pain is moderated by effective coping methods over time rather than chronological age. Another study found that passive coping prior to amputation, particularly the use of catastrophizing, was associated with the development of PLP (Richardson, Glenn, Horgan, & Nurmikko, 2007). Preamputation pain is also a risk factor associated with postoperative PLP.

Treatment of phantom limb pain is difficult, and more efforts recently have been initiated to prevent or minimize the pain associated with PLP. Anticonvulsants such as gabapentin, pregabalin, antidepressants, nonsteroidal anti-inflammatory drugs, and opioid analgesics have varying reports of effectiveness. Regional blocks, intrathecal or epidural opioids, sympathetic blocks, and electrical nerve stimulators have been tried with minimal success. One case report showed pain relief with a multiple spinal cord stimulation system (Coleman & Khodavirdi, 2007).

Efforts to prevent the development of PLP continue to be explored. One case report demonstrated that bupivacaine and clonidine injected preoperatively and infused for 96 hours postoperatively resulted in no report of phantom limb pain. Other efforts to reduce PLP include promotion of positive coping strategies preoperatively.

Central Post-Stroke Pain (CPSP)

Central post-stroke pain (CPSP) is one type of central pain syndrome. Central pain syndrome is a neurological condition caused by damage of the brain, brainstem, or spinal cord (NINDS, 2007). This syndrome can be caused by stroke, multiple sclerosis, tumors, seizures, brain injury, spinal cord injury, or Parkinson's disease. Central pain syndrome may begin shortly after the cause of the injury or can occur several years later as is seen with post-stroke pain. The type of pain experienced is often dependent upon the cause and is typically constant. The pain is moderate to severe in intensity and the patient may experience more than one type of pain sensation. The pain is often made worse by touch, movement emotions, and temperature changes, particularly cold temperatures.

Central stroke pain occurs in 5%–9% of patients who suffer a stroke (Bowsher, 1995). At one time it was thought that this syndrome only occurred in patients with strokes to the thalamus or parietal lobe. A former name for this particular etiology was known as thalamic syndrome. However, this pain has been experienced by patients with strokes from all areas of the brain.

Descriptions of post stroke pain include a burning sensation or a throbbing, pins and needles sensation. The pain typically occurs in large portions of the body, often head to toe. Covering oneself with a blanket or putting on clothing can elicit allodynia, common with post stroke pain. Unique forms of allodynia have been associated with post stroke pain, such as movement, startle, and thermal allodynia (Bowsher, 2005). Patients with central post stroke pain are often unable to differentiate between sharp and dull pain or hot and cold sensations.

Treatment for central post-stroke syndrome centers on the use of neuro-pathic medications such as gabapentin or low-dose tricyclic antidepressant such as amitripyline (Chen, Stitik, Foye, Nadler, & DeLisa, 2002). There has also been some evidence that intrathecal baclofen, an agonist for the gamma aminobutyric acid-B receptor used for controlling spasticity in other syndromes, has benefit for patients with post-stroke central pain (Taira & Hori, 2007). There have also been some suggestions that deep brain stimulation and intrathecal morphine pump has controlled pain associated with central post-stroke pain.

Post-Herpetic Neuralgia

Herpes zoster or shingles is caused by reactivation of the varicella-zoster virus that previously lay dormant in sensory or cranial nerve ganglia (Schmader, 2007). The incidence of herpes zoster is 7.2 to 11.8 per 1,000 population (Schmader, p. 615). Reactivation of the varicella zoster virus evokes an immune and neuronal inflammatory response. As with the varicella zoster virus, patients will experience aching, burning, itching, or tingling pain along the affected dermatone. Once the virus reaches the dermis and epidermis, a unilateral, dermatomal, red, maculopapular rash with vesicles appears. In older adults, atypical rashes may occur, making diagnosis more challenging. Laboratory tests including viral culture, immunofluorescence antigen, or serology are available to differentiate between herpes simplex and herpes zoster. Herpes zoster occurs in the ophthalmic division of the trigeminal nerve in approximately 10%–15% of the cases and can cause ocular complications.

Following the acute phase of herpes zoster, many older adults continue to experience constant or intermittent neuropathic pain or allodynia and develop post-herpetic neuralgia (PHN). PHN is disruptive to daily function and quality of life. In PHN, there is an overall loss of sensory function and signs of denervation. There is a distinct abnormal pattern of cutaneous nerve morphology (Jensen-Dahm, Rice, & Peterson, 2007). It appears that cutaneous afferents remain and peripheral afferents or perhaps their central connections are chronically sensitized (Reda, Rice, Petersen, & Rowbotham, 2006).

There are several treatment options that early in the course of herpes zoster can sometimes minimize the risk of developing PHN. Antiviral medications (acyclovir, famciclovir, and valcyclovir) administered prior to or within 72 hours of the rash appearing have demonstrated a decrease in acute pain and duration of persistent pain. However, even with antivirals early in the course of the disease, there is still a 20%–30% chance of developing PHN

(Schmader, 2007). Use of analgesics in determining the risk for PHN has not been studied.

Acute pain from herpes zoster can be managed with acetaminophen or nonsteroidal anti-inflammatory drugs if the pain is mild. Moderate to severe pain may require a strong opiate for a short term. A neural blockade may also relieve pain if administered early in the course of the disease (Dworkin, Johnson, Breuer, Gnann, Levin, et al., 2007). If the patient develops PHN, a neural block is less likely to be helpful.

The first line of treatment for older adults with post-herpetic neuralgia includes lidocaine patch, gabapentin (Neurontin®), pregabalin (Lyrica®), tricyclic antidepressants, opiates and tramadol. Clinical trials have shown efficacy with these agents. It is noted that topical lidocaine patch, gabapentin and pregabalin have been approved by the FDA for PHN and have resulted in a 30%–60% reduction in pain (Schmader, 2007). Gabapentin can cause sedation, dizziness and edema, therefore if gabapentin is used, it should be given in very low doses beginning at night time and slowly titrated upward. Pregabalin appears to be tolerated fairly well and has a fewer drug interactions. Older adults may benefit from a lower dose (50 mg) three times daily versus 75 mg twice daily. If tricyclic antidepressant medications such as nortriptyline are used, a baseline and follow-up ECG is recommended in older adults (Schmader, 2007). If the older adult has a prolonged QT interval, bundle branch block, or recent myocardial infarction, tricyclic antidepressants are contraindicated. Opioid analgesics and tramadol can be used in the treatment of PHN but the use of these medication need to evaluated individually based on risk versus benefit in the older population. Combination therapy may be indicated if one agent does not adequate relieve the pain of PHN. No data is yet available to indicate whether or not combination therapy has any advantage over monotherapy.

The development of the zoster vaccine (Zostavax®) has been a breakthrough in reducing the incidence of herpes zoster and post-herpetic neuralgia. The zoster vaccine, a live attenuated virus vaccine, is indicated for the prevention of herpes zoster in individuals 60 years of age or older. It is not indicated for the treatment of herpes zoster or PHN. The Shingles Prevention Study, a randomized, double blind, placebo-controlled trial, demonstrated a decreased incidence of herpes zoster by 51.3% and a reduction of PHN by 66.5% (Oxman, Levin, Johnson, Schmader, Straus, et al., 2005). Long-term protective effect currently stands at 4 years. The effectiveness of the vaccine in adults over 80 years of age is unknown as that age group was not included in the trial. The vaccine is contraindicated in acquired immunodeficiency states such as HIV/AIDS, leukemia, lymphoma, or other cancers.

SUMMARY

This chapter describes some of the more common syndromes seen in older adults. Other conditions that cause persistent pain in older adults include chemotherapy-induced pain, painful polyneuropathy, trigeminal neuralgia, chronic regional pain syndrome, greater trochanter pain and gout. Recognizing the origin and generators of pain is crucial to formulating an appropriate treatment plan.

REFERENCES

American Diabetes Association. (2007). Standards of medical care in diabetes. *Diabetic Care, 30,* S4–S41.

American Pain Society. (2005). Guideline for the management of fibromyalgia syndrome pain in adult and children. Retrieved December 29, 2007, from www.ampainsoc.org/pub/fibromyalgia.htm.

Battisti, W. P., Katz, N. P., Weaver, A. L., Matsumoto, A. K., Kivitz, A. J., Polis, A. B., et al. (2004). Pain management in osteoarthritis: a focus on onset of efficacy: A comparison of rofecoxib, celecoxib, acetaminophen, nabumetone across four clinical trials. *Journal of Pain, 5*(9), 511–520.

Bennett, R. (2007). Myofascial pain syndromes and their evaluation. *Best Practices in Research and Clinical Rheumatology, 21*(3), 427–445.

Beyreuther, B. K, Freitag, J., Heers, C., Krebsfanger, N., Scharfenecker, U., & Stohr, T. (2007). Lacosamide: A review of preclinical properties. *CNS Drug Reviews, 13*(1), 21–42.

Blum, D., Biton, V., & Tuchman, M. (2007). Lamotrigine does not alter nerve conduction in patients with diabetic neuropathy. *The Journal of Pain, 8,* S76.

Bowsher, D. (1995). Management of central post-stroke pain. *Postgraduate Medical Journal, 71,* 598–604.

Bowsher, D. (2005). Allodynia in relation to lesion site in central post-stroke pain. *The Journal of Pain, 6*(11), 736–740.

Chen, B., Stitik, T. P., Foye, P. M., Nadler, S. F., & DeLisa, J. A. (2002). Central post-stroke pain syndrome: Yet another use for gabapentin? *American Journal of Physical and Medical Rehabilitation, 81*(9), 718–720.

Coleman, K., & Khodavirdi, A. (2007). Successful treatment of phantom limb pain with Precision™ spinal cord stimulation system: A case report. *The Journal of Pain, 8,* S35.

Davies, C., Davies, A., & Simmons, D. G. (2004). *The trigger point therapy workbook: Your self treatment guide for pain relief* (2nd ed.). Oakland, CA: New Harbinger Publishing.

Davis, J. L, & Smith, R. L. (1999). Painful peripheral diabetic neuropathy treated with venlafaxine HCl extended release capsules. *Diabetes Care, 22,* 1909–1910.

Dworkin, R. H., Johnson, R. W., Breuer, J., Gnann, J. W., Levin, M. J., Backonja, M., et al. (2007). Recommendations for the management of herpes zoster. *Clinical Infectious Diseases, 44,* S1–S26.

Duby, J. J., Campbell, R. K., Setter, S. M., White, J. R., & Rasmussen, K. A. (2004). Diabetic neuropathy: An intensive review. *American Journal of Health-System Pharmacy, 61*(2), 160–173.

Ehde, D., Jensen, M., Williams, R., & Smith, D. (2007). Incidence and severity of pain in he first year after amputation. *The Journal of Pain, 8,* S21.

Endresen, G. K. (2007). Fibromyalgia: A rheumatologic diagnosis? *Rheumatology International, 27,* 999–1004.

Felson, D. T., Niu, J., McClennan, C., Sack, B., Aliabadi, P., Hunter, D. J., et al. (2007). Knee buckling: Prevalence, risk factors, and associated limitations in function. *Annals of Internal Medicine, 147,* 534–540.

Finando, D., & Finando, S. (2005). *Trigger point therapy for myofascial pain: The practice of informed touch.* Rochester, VT: Healing Arts Press.

Ga, H., Choi, J. H., Park, C. H., & Yoon, H. J. (2007). Dry needling of trigger points with and without parasponal needling in myofascial pain syndromes in elderly patients. *Journal of Alternative and Complementary Medicine, 13*(6), 617–624.

Galer, B., Oleka, N., & Gammaitoni, A. (2005). Lidocaine patch 55 improves outcomes for low-back pain and osteoarthritis patients receiving COX-2-selective or traditional NSAID therapy for pain relief. *The Journal of Pain, 6,* S50.

Gammaitoni, A., Oleka, N., & Galer, B. (2005). Lidocaine patch 5% improves outcomes for post-herpetic neuralgia patients receiving COX-2/anti-inflammatory, opioid or adjuvant analgesics. *The Journal of Pain, 6,* 549.

Goldenberg, D. V., Burckhardt, C., & Crofford, L. (2004). Management of fibromyalgia. *Journal of the American Medical Association, 292*(19), 2388–2395.

Gore, M., Brandenburg, N. A., Hoffman, D. L., Tai, K. S., & Stacey, B. (2006). Burden of illness in painful diabetic peripheral neuropathy: The patients' perspective. *The Journal of Pain, 7*(12), 892–900.

Harrington, L., & Schneider, J. I. (2006). Atraumatic joint and limb pain in the elderly. *Emergency Medical Clinics of North America, 24,* 389–412.

Jensen-Dahm, C., Rice, F., & Petersen, K. (2007). Immunochemical characteristics of cutaneous innervations in patients with severe post herpetic neuralgia: a case-control study. *The Journal of Pain, 8,* S29.

Khoromi, S., Patsalides, A., Parada, S., Salehi, V., Meegan, J. M., & Max, M. B. (2005). Topiramate in chronic lumbar radicular pain. *The Journal of Pain, 6*(12), 829–836.

Molton, I., Jensen, M., Ehde, D., & Smith, D. (2007). Phantom limb pain and pain interference in lower extremity amputees: the moderating effects of age. *The Journal of Pain, 8*(4), S63.

National Fibromyalgia Association. (2007). Fibromyalgia. Retrieved December 27, 2007, from www.fmaware.org/PageServer?pagename=fibromayalgia.

National Institute of Neurological Disorders and Stroke (NINDS). (2007). NINDS Central pain syndrome information page. Retrieved December 27, 2007, from www.ninds.nih.gov/disorders/central_pain/central_pain.htm.

Nikolajsen, L., & Jensen, T. S. (2001). Phantom limb pain. *British Journal of Anesthesiology, 87,* 107–116.

Old, J. L., & Calvert, M. (2004). Vertebral compression fractures in the elderly. *American Family Physician, 69,* 111–116.

Oxman, M. N., Levin, M. J., Johnson, G. R, Schmader, K. E., Straus, S. E., Gleb, L. D., et al. (2005). A vaccine to prevent herpes zoster and postherpetic neuralgia in older adults. *New England Journal of Medicine, 352,* 2272–2284.

Podichetty, V. K. (2007). The aging spine: The role of inflammatory mediators in intervertebral disc degeneration. *Cellular and Molecular Biology, 53,* 4–18.

Podichetty, V. K., Mazanec, D. J., & Biscup, R. S. (2003). Chronic non-malignant musculoskeletal pain in older adults: clinical issues and opioid intervention. *Postgraduate Medical Journal, 79*(937), 627–633.

Podichetty, V. K., Spears, J., Isaacs, R. E., Booher, J., & Biscup, R. S. (2006). Complications associated with minimally invasive decompression for lumbar spinal stenosis. *Spinal Disorders and Technology, 19,* 161–166.

Reda, H., Rice, F., Petersen, K., & Rowbotham, M. (2006). Patterns of sensory function and cutaneous innervations in post-herpetic neuralgia. *The Journal of Pain, 7,* S1.

Richardson, C., Glenn, S., Horgan, M., & Nurmikko, T. (2007). A prospective study of actors associated with the presence of phantom limb pain six months after major lower limb amputation in patients with peripheral vascular disease. *The Journal of Pain, 8*(10), 793–801.

Richter, R. W., Portenoy, R., Sharma, U., Lamoreaux, L., Bockbrader, H., & Knapp, L. E. (2005). Relief of painful diabetic peripheral neuropathy with pregabalin: A randomized, placebo controlled trial. *The Journal of Pain, 6*(4), 253–260.

Riley, J. L., Wade, J. B., Robinson, M. E., & Price, D. D. (2000). The stages of pain processing across the adult lifespan. *The Journal of Pain, 1*(2), 162–170.

Schmader, K. (2007). Herpes soster and post herpetic neuralgia in older adults. *Clinical Geriatric Medicine, 23,* 615–632.

Sprenger, T., & Tolle, T. R. (2007). Pain relief by electrostimulation of myofascial trigger points: Peripheral or central mechanisms? *Clinical Journal of Pain, 23,* 638–639.

Starlanyl, D., & Copeland, M. E. (2001). *Fibromyalgia and chronic myofascial pain* (2nd ed.). Oakland, CA: New Harbinger Publications.

Staud, R. (2007). Future perspectives: Pathogenesis of chronic muscle pain. *Best Practices and Research in Clinical Rheumatology, 21*(3), 581–596.

Taira, T., & Hori, T. (2007). Intrathecal baclofen in the treatment of post-stroke central pain, dystonia, and persistent vegetative state. *Acta Neurochirurgica Supplement, 97,* 227–229.

Weiner, D. K. (2007). Office management of chronic pain in elderly. *American Journal of Medicine, 120*(4), 306–315.

Wolfe, F., Smythe, H. A., Yunas, M. B., Bennett, R. M., Bombardier, C., Goldenberg, D. L., et al. (1990). The American College of Rheumatology 1990 criteria for the classification of fibromyalgia: report of the multicenter criteria committee. *Arthritis and Rheumatology, 33*, 160–172.

Wolfe, R., Ross, K., Anderson, J., Russell, I. J., & Hebert, L. (1995). The prevalence and characteristics of fibromyalgia of the general population. *Arthritis and Rheumatology, 38*(1), 19–28.

Wu, E. Q., Birnbaum, H. G., Mareva, M. N., Le, T. K., Robinson, R. L., Rosen, A., et al. (2005). Cost-effectiveness of duloxetine versus routine treatment for U.S. patients with diabetic peripheral neuropathic pain. *The Journal of Pain, 7*(6), 300–407.

CHAPTER 3

Pain Assessment in the Older Adult

Karen S. Feldt

Perhaps the single key to achieving quality pain management for older adults is the accurate assessment of pain. Health professionals who fail to ask about specific pain symptoms or effects place patients at risk for unidentified, misdiagnosed, and under-treated pain. During the late 1990s three key organizations began to focus on improving pain management of patients in a variety of settings. In 1998 the Veteran's Administration started an initiative to make pain the "fifth vital sign" (Department of Veterans Affairs, 2003), and the Joint Commission on Accreditation of Health Care Organizations followed suit in 1999, settings standards for assessing and managing pain (JCAHO, 2006). Finally, a committee commissioned by the Centers for Medicare and Medicaid examined the quality indicators in long-term care facilities and made recommendations to include pain as a quality indicator (Berg, Mor, Morris, Murphy, Moore, et al., 2002). With these initiatives demanding better pain assessment, researchers have worked to develop appropriate assessment tools that address the unique issues of the older population. Instruments that can objectively measure pain in a standardized fashion are critical in the initiation of pain management strategies and the ongoing evaluation of the efficacy of that pain management. This chapter critiques the literature regarding existing pain assessment instruments identified as useful for older adults and examines emerging research on tools recommended for assessing specific types of pain (neuropathic) and for assessing pain in specific populations of older adults (nonverbal cognitively impaired older adults).

COMPREHENSIVE PAIN ASSESSMENT INSTRUMENTS

A comprehensive assessment of pain should include an interview that allows the older adult to tell their pain story. The waxing and waning nature of chronic pain, with an overlap of acute pain problems, in older adults can create difficulties if the person is simply asked to rate their pain as if it is a single event. Busy clinicians often obtain only severity ratings and locations of the pain, a small part of the pain assessment picture. Clinicians must believe the patient's pain story and ratings of severity, since patient report is the gold standard of pain assessment (McCaffery & Pasero, 1999). Health care providers should allow time for the older person to talk about the quality and character of the pain. Pain described as "aching" or "pressure" (likely nociceptive pain) may be treated quite differently than pain that is described as "burning" or "shooting" (likely neuropathic pain). Patients should be encouraged to give descriptions of when the pain occurs and whether certain activities make this pain worse. Identifying specific patterns and changes in the intensity of pain can influence how and when pain treatments should be scheduled to manage pain.

Comprehensive pain assessment must include questions about whether and/or how this pain affects the person's physical and social functioning. What impact does the pain have on daily activities, mood, outlook, or functions? A thorough understanding of the types and frequency of pain medications, the efficacy of those treatments, or the use of other nonpharmacological treatments should be explored. It is not unusual for patients or nursing staff to demand stronger pain medications for a patient when the current prescription has not even been given routinely or at an adequate dose. Finally, the clinician should assess the patient's understanding of the pain and their expectations or goals for treatment (AGS Panel on Chronic Pain in Older Persons, 1998; AGS Panel on Persistent Pain in Older Persons, 2002; Herr, 2004; McCaffery & Pasero, 1999). There are patients that are unable to provide a self-report of pain. Family members or staff who know the patient well may be able to identify changes in functioning, behavior, or mood that could indicate pain. Substituting proxy reports of pain may be helpful but may also lead to inaccurate conclusions. Several studies have demonstrated that when compared with patient ratings of pain, nurses' or nursing assistants' estimates of pain are not congruent, either underestimating or overestimating pain in older adults (Bergh & Sjostrom, 1999; Engle, Graney, & Chan, 2001; Horgas & Dunn, 2001; Scherder & van Manen, 2005; Weiner, Petersen, & Keefe, 1999).

The McGill pain questionnaire (MPQ), a widely used comprehensive pain assessment tool developed by Melzack (1975), includes a listing of 78 words that have been categorized into 20 groups, a body drawing, and a pain intensity subscale, which represent the sensory, affective, and evaluative dimensions of pain. Although designed to be comprehensive in scope, the tool does not assess the impact of pain on functional activities. The time required to complete this instrument makes it better suited to a comprehensive pain center than a busy clinic or institutional setting. The visual and hearing impairments in older subjects could interfere with comprehension and lengthen the time required for pain assessment using this tool. Vocabulary comprehension problems may also limit its usefulness in patients with lower educational levels or cognitive impairment. However, Gagliese and Melzack (1997) report that older persons have no difficulty with the MPQ and are likely to use *more* verbal descriptors of pain, rather than fewer verbal descriptors as used by younger patients, a finding supported by other pain researchers (Ferrell, Ferrell, & Osterweil, 1990). The Present Pain Intensity (PPI) subscale (rating of "no pain," "mild," "discomforting," "distressing," "horrible," and "excruciating") of the MPQ has been used successfully with older adults, including those with cognitive impairment. The vocabulary words in this instrument are more complex as compared with the Verbal Descriptor Scale and may appeal to older adults with higher educational levels. However, two-thirds (60%–67%) of cognitively impaired older adults in nursing home and hospital studies were able to rate their pain on this subscale (Kaasalainen & Crook, 2004; Ferrell, Ferrell, & Rivera, 1995; Mosier, Nusser-Gerlach, Manz, & Bergstrom, 1998).

The Geriatric Pain Measure is an instrument that was developed to capture more of the functional components of chronic pain (Ferrell, Stein, & Beck, 2000). It includes the functional and social impact as well as the intensity of pain in geriatric patients. The instrument has five clusters of components, including, pain intensity, disengagement, pain with ambulation, pain with strenuous activities, and pain with other activities. It is a 24-item questionnaire that has several questions in a yes/no format for ease of use with older adults and also has a numeric rating scale for current pain and pain within the past week. It has been piloted in 176 older adults with a history of chronic pain who were clinic patients at a veterans' facility. The instrument total score shows significant correlations ($r = .62$, $P<.0000$) with the McGill Total Score and with the Present Pain Intensity subscale ($.54$, $P<.0000$). Test–retest reliability was conducted on a subset of subjects 48 to 72 hours apart with a strong correlation of $r = .90$ ($P<.0000$), and item agreement on the dichotomous items with kappa of 0.597 (Ferrell, Stein, & Beck, 2000). The measure was simplified to a 17-item questionnaire for use in a sample of nursing home residents, with good internal consistency (Cronbach's $\alpha = 0.87$–0.91) and test–retest reliability ($r = .74$–$.80$). Concurrent validity, a correlation of the tool score with the number of chronic pain–associated diagnoses, was poor for residents in the low to moderate cognitive status group ($r = .25$, $p = .18$), but was somewhat better for residents in the moderate to high cognitive status group ($r = .42$, $p = .02$). Difficulties with the instrument in cognitively impaired older adults are not surprising, given the need to remember whether pain is a problem during daily activities, but modifications have made the instrument potentially useful for staff working with older adults in long-term care settings (Fisher, Burgio, Thorn, & Hardin, 2006).

Pain Intensity/Severity Assessment Instruments

Pain severity instruments provide a brief measure of current or recent pain intensity. Although these instruments are not comprehensive in their very nature, they do provide a quick objective measure of evaluating pain severity, measuring treatment efficacy, and general patient comfort. This section will review several instruments that can be used to assess pain severity or intensity in older adults who have the cognitive skills necessary to understand and rate their own pain. Although there are other instruments, this section will review the Verbal Descriptor Scale (Exhibit 3.1), the Verbal Numeric Scale (Exhibit 3.2), the Visual Analog Scale (Exhibit 3.3), and the Faces Pain Scale.

The pain intensity tool most preferred by the older subjects is the Verbal Descriptor Scale (VDS) (Herr & Mobily, 1993; Herr, Spratt, Mobily, & Richardson, 2004; Jones, Fink, Hutt, Vojir, Pepper, et al., 2005; Taylor, Harris, Epps, & Herr, 2005). The VDS is a variation of the Present Pain Intensity subscale developed by Melzack (1975). Pain severity descriptions are in simple language, "no pain," "slight pain," to "extreme pain," and "pain as bad as it could be." When used in large-print format (Exhibit 3.1), older adults who are hearing impaired can simply point to the words that best describe their

---

EXHIBIT 3.1 VERBAL DESCRIPTOR SCALE

_____	(10)	PAIN AS BAD AS IT COULD BE
_____	(8-9)	EXTREME PAIN
_____	(6-7)	SEVERE PAIN
_____	(4-5)	MODERATE PAIN
_____	(2-3)	MILD PAIN
_____	(1)	SLIGHT PAIN
_____	(0)	NO PAIN

pain. The VDS has been highly correlated ($r = .86$ to $.96$) with other measures of pain intensity (Herr & Mobily, 1993; Herr, Spratt, Mobily, & Richardson, 2004; Taylor, Harris, Epps, & Herr, 2005). This tool is understood by older adults with lower education levels and has a low failure rate (2%). In studies of assisted living and nursing home residents, between 52% and 97% of residents were able to successfully use the scale (Jones et al., 2005; Kaasalainen & Crook, 2004; Taylor, Harris, Epps, & Herr, 2005). The VDS was printed in large bold print and successfully completed by 73% of hospitalized cognitively impaired older adults following hip fracture surgery (Feldt, Ryden, & Miles, 1998). Although the scale is limited, in that it measures only a single dimension of pain (pain severity or intensity) its simplicity makes it easy for busy clinicians to use in routine assessments of pain and evaluations of pain treatment outcomes.

The most commonly used pain assessment is a simple verbal numeric scale (VNS). The patient is asked verbally: "On a scale of 0 to 10, with 0 being no pain and 10 being the worst pain you can imagine, how would you rank your pain?" (Exhibit 3.2). Although this scale is widely used, there are problems with this use of this scale in the older population. Studies have shown that cognitively intact older adults and 50%–70% of mildly cognitively impaired older adults are able to understand the scale (Jones et al., 2005; Kaasalainen & Crook, 2004; Taylor, Harris, Epps, & Herr, 2005). However, research comparing scales identifies that older women and older adults with lower educational levels (high school or less) do not prefer to use this scale (Taylor, Harris, Epps, & Herr, 2005). In a large study of 1,182 nursing home residents, only 29% identified this scale as their preferred tool for rating pain (Jones et al., 2005). The tool has been found to be problematic for older adults with cognitive impairment because of the need to abstract a sensation concept (usually described by older adults as a word, e.g., "mild," "pressing," "severe") into a numeric concept. One-third of nursing home residents in general (not just cognitively impaired) were unable to use the 0–10 scale (Weiner, Ladd, Pieper, & Keefe, 1995), and less than half of cognitively impaired residents were able to respond to this scale (Ferrell, Ferrell, & Rivera, 1995). Some researchers have

---

EXHIBIT 3.2 VERBAL NUMERIC SCALE

"On a scale of 0 to 10, with 0 being no pain and 10 being the worst pain you can imagine, how would you rank your pain?"

recommended changes to collapse the NRS to a five-point scale (0–4) to reduce complexity, or to assess older adults using the scale substituting the word "discomfort" for pain (Fulmer, Mion, & Bottrel, 1996; Morrison, Ahronheim, Morrison, Darling, Baskin, et al., 1998). For patients or residents who are able to use the scale, concurrent validity of the NRS is excellent, with correlations of .81 to .93 between the NRS and the Verbal Descriptor Scale (VDS) or the visual analogue scale (VAS) (Taylor & Herr, 2003; Stuppy, 1998).

The VAS is a simple 100 mm line with anchored words at either end of the line identifying "no pain" and "the worst pain possible" (Exhibit 3.3). Older adults are asked to place a mark on a line to indicate the degree of pain experienced. The American Geriatrics Society Chronic Pain Management Guidelines (AGS Panel on Chronic Pain in Older Persons, 1998) recommend modifying the VAS by adding anchored pain descriptors along the scale as a guide to older adults (Exhibit 3.3). In its original format, the tool has a failure rate of between 6.7% and 19.1% for older adults (Herr, Spratt, Mobily, & Richardson, 2004; Herr & Mobily, 1993). Although highly correlated with other measures of pain intensity, retest reliability within 5 mm of the previous mark is poor (DeLoach, Higgins, Caplan, & Stiff, 1998; Herr & Mobily, 1993). Only 44% of nursing home residents, 27% to 79% of hospitalized older adults, and 41% to 76% of community-dwelling older adults with cognitive impairment were able to successfully understand and complete this scale (Ferrell, Ferrell, & Rivera, 1995; Krulewitch, London, Skakel, Lundstedt, Thomason, et al. 2000; Pautex, Harrmann, LeLous, Fabjan, Michel, et al., 2005). A recent study reported that the VAS was the least preferred of the pain rating scales tested in community-dwelling older adults, with only 10.9% of the participants selecting it as preferred (Herr, Spratt, Mobily, & Richardson, 2004).

The Faces Pain Scale (FPS) is a series of facial expressions representing different degrees of pain intensity (Bieri, Reeve, Champion, Addicoat, & Ziegler,

---

EXHIBIT 3.3 THE VISUAL ANALOG SCALE

This scale is measured to be exactly 100 mm long

No pain   Worst pain

|_____|

Or, as modified by the AGS guidelines with more anchor words:

No pain   Mild pain   Moderate pain   Severe pain   Extreme pain

|_____|_____|_____|_____|

1990). Originally developed for use with children, the scale has recently been tested with cognitively intact older adults as well as older adults with dementia. The scale has had mixed findings by researchers, with some finding it well comprehended and finding it to have strong construct validity and test–retest reliability ($r = 0.94$, $p = .01$) (Stuppy, 1998; Scherder, Bouma, Slaets, Ooms, Ribbe, et al., 2001; Herr, Spratt, Mobily, & Richardson, 2004; Kim & Buschmann, 2006), while others have found it to be less strongly related to ratings on other pain scales, poorly understood, and less reliable (Kaasalainen & Crook, 2004; Herr, Spratt, Mobily, & Richardson, 2004; Wynne, Ling, & Remsburg, 2000). The instrument receives inconsistent marks in terms of preference for use by older adults compared with other pain scales. The FPS was the preferred tool for only 12% to 19% of the subjects tested in three different studies (Herr, Spratt, Mobily, & Richardson, 2004; Kaasalainen & Crook, 2004; Jones et al., 2005) but was preferred by 54% of minority older adults in another study (Ware, Epps, Herr, & Packard, 2006).

Kaasalainen and Crook (2004) reported that cognitively intact nursing home residents had some difficulty choosing the correct face that depicted the most and least pain and that fewer than one-third of the residents in their study could place the faces in the correct order from least to worst pain. Several studies have identified that the Faces Pain Scale is not well understood by cognitively impaired older adults: 30% to 60% of impaired older adults were unable to appropriately understand and use the tool (Kaasalainen & Crook, 2004; Scherder & Bouma, 2000; Jones et al., 2005). A study that used the Wong-Baker Faces scale (a different set of simple faces) found that only one-third of the cognitively impaired nursing home residents tested to successfully use that scale (Wynne, Ling, & Remsburg, 2000). Researchers' anecdotal comments on this scale indicate that, in its current form it is problematic in the older adult population. One researcher writes: "The FPS...is a poorer choice because even the cognitively intact older adult demonstrated some difficulty with the interpretation of the scale. For example, some residents stated that the last face on the scale was 'laughing at them' when it was intended to display a face full of pain at the highest level" (Kaasalainen & Crook, 2004). Given these difficulties, this scale is not recommended as a first choice for pain intensity measures in older adults.

Pain Assessment Instruments for Special Populations

Older Adults With Neuropathic Pain

As indicated in previous chapters, persistent pain can generally be classified into two distinct types of pain, with differing pain mechanisms and presentation of symptoms: nociceptive pain and neuropathic pain. Because neuropathic pain is treated in a very different way than nociceptive pain, it is essential that health care professionals be adept at assessment of neuropathic pain signs and symptoms. Simple pain intensity tools as described in the previous section do not provide adequate assessment for patients with neuropathic pain. There are a few emerging pain assessment instruments designed and tested for use in identifying patients with neuropathic pain. Two of these assessment instruments will be discussed here: the Leeds Assessment of Neuropathic Symptoms and Signs (LANSS Pain Scale) (Bennett, 2001) and the Neuropathic Pain Questionnaire (Krause & Backonja, 2003).

The Leeds Assessment of Neuropathic Symptoms and Signs (LANSS) pain scale was developed by Bennett (2001) as an instrument that distinguishes neuropathic symptoms and signs from nociceptive pain. The work done in developing this instrument identified specific descriptors that are significantly associated with neuropathic pain as compared with nociceptive pain. The scale includes two components, a pain questionnaire that asks five questions using the neuropathic-specific descriptors (for example, question 1 asks: Does your pain feel like strange, unpleasant sensation in your skin? Words like pricking, tingling, and pins and needles might describe these sensations). Each question receives a dichotomous score, although the weighting of the yes/no score varies for each item. The second component of the scale requires skin sensitivity testing for the presence of allodynia and altered pin-prick threshold.

In a study of 40 patients recruited from a chronic pain clinic, the LANSS pain scale was able to correctly identify 82% of the patients (positive predictive value) and had a negative predictive value of 84%. Internal consistency of the instrument was good with a Cronbach's alpha of 0.74, and the investigator/clinician agreement on the pain type and items on the scale were good with kappa values between 0.6 and 0.88 (Bennett, 2001). The authors then modified the scale into a self-report version (the S-LANSS) and sent it out in survey form to 310 patients, half of whom were patients from a pain clinic and the other half from a general practice setting. The S-LANSS demonstrated a sensitivity of 74% to 78%, and good internal consistency (Cronbach's alpha .80) and convergent validity with the NPS (Bennett, Smith, Torrance, & Potter, 2005). In another study, the researchers showed that there were significant differences between the S-LANSS and the Neuropathic Pain Questionnaire, but that higher scores on either of the instruments are indicative of a greater clinical certainty that the patient has neuropathic pain (Bennett, Smith, Torrance, & Lee, 2006). The original LANSS assessment instrument is relatively simple to use but does requires some equipment (cotton wool for the allodynia testing and a needle for the altered pin-prick threshold), and some relative experience in examination skills, especially neurological exam skills. The S-LANSS as a self-report instrument appears to be easily understood by adult patients; however, it has not been tested in older adults or frail older adults.

The Neuropathic Pain Questionnaire is a self-report instrument that uses descriptors common in persons with neuropathic pain (Krause & Backonja, 2003). This instrument does not provide a pain score that can be used to determine efficacy of treatment, but rather is a complex scoring method to determine if the patient most likely has neuropathic pain. Initial testing of the instrument was conducted on 528 persistent pain patients from several clinics within a university setting, 149 of these known to have neuropathic pain. The mean age of subjects participating was 47 years. The instrument is a 12-item questionnaire that requires the patient to rate each of the descriptors on a scale of 1 to 100. Older adults expressed difficulty in other studies when asked to complete visual analog scales that had ranges of 1 to 100 (Krulewitch et al., 2000; Pautex et al., 2005). This instrument has not yet been studied in large populations of older adults but may have similar problems, given that all 12 items require a rating score in a range of 1 to 100. The instrument has a 66% sensitivity and 74% specificity. Internal consistency on the original 32-item questionnaire was 0.95; however, the internal consistency on the final 12-item tool is not reported. Clinicians using the tool are required to complete a calculated score, multiplying the patient's rating by a specific coefficient for each item and summing the scores with a constant coefficient. The final score provides a discriminant function score that is either predictive of neuropathic pain or predictive of non-neuropathic pain (Krause & Backonja, 2003).

Older Adults With Arthritis

There are several measures that have been developed to specifically address the issues of pain in older adults with arthritic conditions. Although these measures are multidimensional, assessing the full impact of arthritis on the individual's functional status, mood, and social activity, each of them has pain subscales that are designed to assess pain within the context of this disease. The Arthritis Impact Measurement Scale (AIMS) is a scale that was designed specifically to assess the health of older adults with arthritis and other rheumatic diseases (Meenan, Gertman, & Mason, 1980). The authors revised and expanded this instrument in 1992 (AIMS2) to include four subscales: physical function, symptoms, affect, and social function. The symptom subscale of the AIMS2 is the scale that addresses pain. Patients are asked to rate their symptoms on a five-point Likert scale as to how much of the time in the past four weeks they were bothered by: severe pain from arthritis; two or more painful joints at one time; morning stiffness that lasts more than one hour; pain that makes it difficult to go to sleep (Ren, Kazis, & Meenan, 1999). Internal consistency for the pain subscale has been measured to range between 0.74 to 0.80 (Ren, Kazis, & Meenan, 1999).

Some difficulties with the AIMS are that it requires the older adult to think over a relatively long period of time (four weeks) and identify a single response on a Likert scale to the item requested. This would be problematic for older adults with memory problems. Older adults often "tell the story" of their pain and its daily fluctuations, but they sometimes have a difficult time specifically identifying a single item on a Likert scale.

The Western Ontario and McMaster University Osteoarthritis Index was also developed to provide a comprehensive assessment of the impact of arthritis (Bellamy, 1989). The index uses a Likert scale or visual analogue scale format to measure items in the subscales. The pain subscale has five items that ask about pain severity during common daily activities: walking on a flat surface, going up and down stairs, sleeping, sitting or lying down, and standing. Cronbach's alpha for the WOMAC scale is 0.85, and test re–test reliability of the WOMAC is good (0.82 to 0.86) (Bellamy, 1989). The scale has been interpreted into several languages, among them Dutch, Spanish, Turkish, and Japanese. A study by Tsai and Tak demonstrated that even cognitively impaired elders with scores on the MMSE between 11 and 24 were able to complete the WOMAC with good reliability (Tsai & Tak, 2003).

Cognitively Impaired Nonverbal Older Adults

Assessment of pain in cognitively impaired older adults is complicated by the gradual global cognitive losses, including short-term memory skills, impaired abstraction, impaired verbal skills (especially naming and word-finding problems), and eventually loss of verbalizations (U.S. Department of Health and Human Services, 2005). Nursing staff may discount complaints because of inconsistency or lack of reliability of patient report. Researchers agree that simple pain intensity instruments can be used while verbal skills are intact (Fisher et al., 2006; Jones et al., 2005; Kaasalainen & Crook, 2004). However, once verbal skills are lost, observational scales and surrogate reports become necessary as determinants of pain (Herr, Bjoro, & Decker, 2006). The most comprehensive review of all the instruments developed for pain assessment of nonverbal cognitively impaired older adults was conducted by Herr and colleagues (2006). These authors provide an in-depth critique and analysis of 10 instruments recommended for assessment of pain in nonverbal older adults.

The Mayday Fund provides electronic access to a more detailed critique of each instrument at: http://www.cityofhope.org/prc/elderly.asp.

Given page constraints, this section will describe and review five assessment instruments that attend to behavioral cues indicative of the presence of pain. Three instruments that are designed to assess pain in the nonverbal population are not reviewed here for specific reasons. The Face Legs Cry and Consolability (FLACC) Pain Assessment tool was originally designed to assess pain in young children, and the tool items are not conceptually appropriate for use in cognitively impaired older adults (Manworren & Hynan, 2003; Baiardi, Parzuchowski, & Kosik, 2002; Herr, Bjoro, & Decker, 2006). The Assessment of Discomfort in Dementia (ADD) protocol is not reviewed because it is a systematic evaluative approach to behavior change that might indicate pain, rather than a specific pain assessment instrument (Kovach, Noonan, Griffie, Muchka, & Weissman, 1999). The Doloplus 2 is not reviewed because of the lack of English-based testing and the interpretation of the psychosocial items within the tool (Wary & Doloplus, 1999; Hølen, Saltvedt, Fayers, Bjørnnes, Stenseth, et al., 2005).

Discomfort in Dementia of the Alzheimer's type (DS-DAT). One of the initial scales developed and tested for measuring discomfort in non-communicative patients with advanced Alzheimer's type dementia is the Discomfort in Dementia of the Alzheimer's type (DS-DAT) (Hurley, Volicer, Hanrahan, Houde, & Volicer, 1992). Discomfort, defined by these researchers as a negative emotional and/or physical state subject to variation in magnitude in response to internal or environmental conditions, differs somewhat from the concept of pain (Herr, Bjoro, & Decker, 2006). The (DS-DAT) scale includes nine items, two positive and seven negative: noisy breathing, negative vocalization, content facial expression, sad facial expression, frightened facial expression, frown, relaxed body language, tense body language, and fidgeting. Observers scored each item on a continuous scale from absent (0) to extreme (100) based on the presence of the defining characteristics. Although initial testing showed good inter-rater reliability (.86 to .98) and tool reliability (Cronbach's alpha .86 to .89), the tool was used on a mostly male (90%), fairly small sample (N = 82) (Hurley, Volicer, Hanrahan, Houde, & Volicer, 1992). One of the items, noisy breathing, could be attributed to medical conditions such as an upper respiratory tract infection or chronic obstructive pulmonary disease. Facial expressions of discomfort may differ by gender and culture.

Researchers using the DS-DAT have identified difficulty with inter-rater reliability for specific items (relaxed body language, sad facial expression, and frown) and modified the tool to improve the reliability (Miller, Neelon, Dalton, Ng'andu, Bailey, et al., 1996). These researchers identified that the

DS-DAT is not "user friendly" for routine nursing care because of the in-depth training required to obtain accurate, reliable ratings. However, research assistants believed the DS-DAT is useful in reflecting relative changes in hospitalized patients' discomfort and has been useful in detecting changes in comfort levels in nursing home populations (Miller et al., 1996; Kovach, Weissman, Griffe, Matson, & Muchka, 1999).

While the DS-DAT is a reliable tool for measuring discomfort in cognitively impaired older adults, it requires extensive training for use and is limited to observations of pain at rest. These issues may limit its usefulness in a clinical setting (Herr, Bjoro, & Decker, 2006).

PAINAD scale. This pain scale is an adaptation of the DS-DAT and the Face Legs Cry and Consolability (FLACC) pain assessment tool (Manworren & Hynan, 2003; Warden, Hurley, & Volicer, 2003). This was developed by researchers to simplify the DS-DAT into a format that might be more easily used by staff. The five items on the scale: breathing, negative vocalization, facial expression, body language, and consolability are rated by observers on a three-point scale of intensity (0 to 2), providing an overall possible score of 10. The instrument's internal consistency as measured by a Cronbach's alpha is $0.5 - 0.65$, and the inter-rater reliability is reported at 0.82–0.97 (Warden, Hurley, & Volicer, 2003). The PAINAD scale correlates was with the Pain VAS, the DS-DAT, and the Discomfort VAS, ($r = 0.75, 0.76, 0.76$ respectively); however, given that several of the items on the PAINAD are directly taken from the DS-DAT, this finding is not surprising.

One of the items on the instrument is consolability, which is a response to an intervention by a nurse, rather than a specific patient behavior. Since this concept is not well tested in its link to pain in cognitively impaired older adults, it is difficult to support its use without further testing (Herr, Bjoro, & Decker, 2006). Another concern about the PAINAD scale is that the authors structured the scale to offer a 0–10 score, similar to the 0–10 Verbal Numeric Rating Scale. Unfortunately, the research does not support a direct 1:1 correlation of the ratings on a behavioral scale with those self ratings on a Verbal Numeric Scale. A behavioral tool score cannot be directly compared with the severity or intensity of pain on self rating (Herr, Bjoro, & Decker, 2006; Herr, Coyne, Key, Manworren, McCaffery, et al., 2006). If nurses expect to see higher scores before treating, the instrument may be misleading.

Checklist of Nonverbal Pain Indicators. Feldt (2000) developed a Checklist of Nonverbal Pain Indicators (CNPI) to identify pain in nonverbal cognitively impaired older adults (Exhibit 3.4). This scale was initially used in hospitalized older adults with hip fractures (Feldt, Ryden, & Miles, 1998), but has also been tested in older adults in long-term care facilities (Feldt & Finch, 2002;

Nygaard & Jarland, 2006; Jones et al., 2005). The instrument includes six items: vocal complaints (expression of pain in moans, groans, grunts, cries, gasps, or sighs); facial grimaces/winces (furrowed brow, narrowed eyes, tightened lips, jaw drop, clenched teeth, or distorted expressions); bracing (clutching or grasping side rails, bed, tray table, or affected area during movement); restlessness (constant or intermittent shifting of position, rocking, intermittent or constant hand motions, inability to keep still); rubbing (massaging affected area); and vocal complaints (words expressing discomfort or pain, "ouch," "that hurts"; cursing during movement, exclamations of protest: "stop," "that's enough"). Inter-rater reliability for the CNPI showed 93% agreement on the dichotomous checklist items; Kappa statistic = 0.625 to 0.819 (p = .019 to .0057) for the behaviors observed using master's-prepared nurses (Feldt, 2000) and lower inter-rater reliability Kappa statistic = 0.45 to 0.69 in a study using staff nurses in long-term care (Nygaard & Jarland, 2006). Initial testing on 87 hip fracture patients revealed an alpha coefficient of .54 for observations using the scale while the patient was at rest, and an alpha coefficient of .64 for observations of patients during movement.

Test–retest ratings in other studies were moderate to good (0.45–0.69) (Nygaard & Jarland, 2006). Jones and colleagues (2005) found that the instrument had better specificity than sensitivity; for residents not reporting pain, 85% had no observable pain behaviors, but for residents reporting pain, 53% had at least one observable behavior. The scale has been significantly modestly correlated with the VDS (CNPI at rest with VDS, Spearman correlation r_s = .372, p = .001; CNPI with movement with VDS, r_s = .428, p < .0001) (Feldt, 2000) and was more strongly correlated with the VAS in another study (Spearman correlation r_s = 0.69 to 0.88) (Nygaard & Jarland, 2006).

Overall the CNPI is a brief instrument that may be easily used in clinical settings. However, given the low frequency of pain behaviors on the CNPI in persons who otherwise report pain, a significant amount of pain may go undetected and untreated if this instrument is used in isolation or if staff nurses assume that several behaviors must be present for pain to be treated (Jones et al., 2005).

NOPPAIN. The Noncommunicative Patient's Pain Assessment Instrument (NOPPAIN) is an instrument developed for use by nursing assistants in providing information to long-term care nursing staff on potential pain in cognitively impaired older adults (Snow, Weber, O'Malley, Cody, Beck, et al., 2004). Similar to the CNPI, pain is assessed at rest and with movement, when residents are doing common care tasks. The instrument has four main sections: care conditions during which pain behaviors are observed (bathing,

EXHIBIT 3.4 CHECKLIST OF NONVERBAL PAIN INDICATORS

Score 0 if not observed, 1 if observed

	With movement	Rest
1. Vocal complaints: Nonverbal (Expression of pain, not in words: moans, groans, grunts, cries, gasps, sighs)	_____	_____
2. Facial Grimaces/Winces (Furrowed brow, narrowed eyes, tightened lips, jaw drop, clenched teeth, distorted expressions).	_____	_____
3. Bracing (Clutching or holding onto side rails, bed, tray table, or affected area during movement)	_____	_____
4. Restlessness (Constant or intermittent shifting of position, rocking, intermittent or constant hand motions, inability to keep still)	_____	_____
5. Rubbing: (Massaging affected area) (In addition, record verbal complaints).	_____	_____
6. Vocal complaints: Verbal (Words expressing discomfort or pain, "ouch," "that hurts"; cursing during movement, or exclamations of protest "stop," "that's enough.")	_____	_____
subscore	_____	_____
Total Score	_____	

dressing, transfers); six items identifying the presence or absence of pain be-haviors (pain words, pain noises, pain faces, bracing, rubbing, and restless-ness); a six-point Likert scale rating of pain intensity, and a pain thermometer for rating pain intensity. Initial testing of agreement between nursing assistant ratings and pain levels portrayed in videos showed a weighted kappa of 0.87. The instrument has not been extensively tested for reliability and validity and there is no guide for interpreting scoring.

Although this tool has potential for use in long-term care facilities, there is no data testing the instrument in real clinical settings. The testing of the tool with an artificial situation on video (acting out a painful situation), rather than with real patients in real settings, limits the ability to give strong support for the use of this tool (Zwakhalen, Hamers, Abu-Saad, & Berger, 2006).

Pain Assessment Checklist of Seniors with Limited Ability to Communicate (PACSLAC). This pain assessment instrument is an observational tool in the form of a checklist with 60 items, all scored on a dichotomous scale (present/absent). The tool has four subscales: facial expressions (13 items), activity/body movements (20 items), social/personality/mood (12 items), and physi-ological indicators/eating and sleeping changes/vocal behaviors (15 items). Internal consistency analysis for the scale as a whole are good (Cronbach's alpha = 0.82 to .92), but the internal consistency of the subscales is moderate (Cronbach's alpha = .55 to .73). Unfortunately, the initial internal consistency was based on remembered events, not current active evaluation of present pain. It is questionable whether caregivers can accurately remember how they would respond to all of 60 items when recalling a pain event (Herr, Bjoro, & Decker, 2006; Zwakhalen, Hamers, & Berger, 2006). No inter-rater reliability or factor analysis of the scale is available.

This tool is potentially a useful clinical checklist that includes many more subtle aspects of pain behavior, as compared with many of the other tools identified above. The tool needs testing on larger samples with inter-rater reli-ability and validity testing to confirm its integrity and usefulness in clinical situations.

SUMMARY

Assessment of pain is essential for the evaluation of comfort and pain management strategies. Recommendations regarding appropriate pain as-sessment instruments for older adults have been established by intensive reviews and pain guidelines (AGS Panel on Chronic Pain in Older Persons, 1998; Herr, Bjoro, & Decker, 2006; Herr et al., 2006; Zwakhalen, Hamers,

Abu-Saad, & Berger, 2006). Ongoing research should establish clear inter-pretation of nonverbal pain assessment instruments. Future instrument re-finement and development should enhance our ability to provide better pain management for all older adults.

REFERENCES

American Geriatrics Society Panel on Chronic Pain in Older Persons. (1998). The management of pain in older persons. *Journal of the American Geriatrics Society, 46,* 635–651.

American Geriatrics Society Panel on Persistent Pain in Older Persons. (2002). The management of persistent pain in older persons. *Journal of the American Geriatrics Society, 50* (Suppl.), 205–234.

Baiardi, J., Parzuchowski, J. & Kosik, C. (2002, September). *Examination of the reliability of the FLACC pain assessment tool with cognitively impaired elderly.* Presentation at the National Conference of Gerontological Nurse Practitioners, Chicago, IL.

Bellamy, N. (1989). Pain assessment in osteoarthritis: Experience with the WOMAC osteoarthritis index. *Seminars in Arthritis and Rheumatism, 18*(4 Suppl. 2), 14–17.

Bennett, M. (2001). The LANSS Pain Scale: The Leeds assessment of neuropathic symptoms and signs. *Pain, 92*(1–2), 147–157.

Bennett, M., Smith, B. H., Torrance, L., & Lee, A. J. (2006). Can pain be more or less neuropathic? Comparison of symptom assessment tools with ratings of certainty by clinicians. *Pain, 122*(3), 289–294.

Bennett, M., Smith, B. H., Torrance, N., & Potter, J. (2005). The S-LANSS score for identifying pain of predominantly neuropathic origin: Validation for use in clinical and postal research. *Journal of Pain, 6*(3), 149–158.

Berg, K., Mor, V., Morris, J., Murphy, K. M., Moore, T., & Harris, Y. (2002). Identification and evaluation of existing nursing home quality indicators. *Health Care Financing Review, 23*(4), 19–36.

Bergh, I., & Sjostrom, B. (1999). A comparative study of nurses' and elderly patients' ratings of pain and pain tolerance. *Journal of Gerontological Nursing, 25*(5), 30–36.

Bieri, D., Reeve, R., Champion, D., Addicoat, L., & Ziegler, J. (1990). The Faces Pain Scale for the self-assessment of the severity of pain experienced by children: Development, initial validation, and preliminary investigation for ratio scale properties. *Pain, 41,* 139–150.

DeLoach, L. J., Higgins, M. S., Caplan, A. B., & Stiff, J. L. (1998). The visual analog scale in the immediate postoperative period: Intrasubject variability and correlation with a numeric scale. *Anesthesia Analgesia, 86,* 102–106.

Department of Veterans Affairs. (2003). VHA directive on pain management, VHA directive 2003–021. Retrieved December 2, 2007, from http://www1va.gov/pain_manage ment/docs/VHAPainDirective_03.pdf.

Engle, V. F., Graney, M. J., & Chan, A. (2001). Accuracy and bias of licensed practical nurse and nursing assistant ratings of nursing home residents' pain. *Journal of Gerontology Series A Biological Sciences and Medical Sciences, 56*(7), M405–M411.

Feldt, K. S. (2000). Checklist of non-verbal pain indicators. *Pain Management Nursing, 1*(1), 13–21.

Feldt, K. S., & Finch, M. (2002). Older adults with hip fractures: Treatment of pain following hospitalization. *Journal of Gerontological Nursing, 28*(8), 27–35.

Feldt, K. S., Ryden, M. B., & Miles, S. (1998). Treatment of pain in cognitively impaired compared with cognitively intact older patients with hip fracture. *Journal of the American Geriatrics Society, 46*, 1079–1085.

Ferrell, B. A., Ferrell, B. R., & Osterweil, D. (1990). Pain in the nursing home. *Journal of the American Geriatrics Society, 38*, 409–414.

Ferrell, B. A., Ferrell, B. R., & Rivera, L. (1995). Pain in cognitively impaired nursing home patients. *Journal of Pain and Symptom Management, 10*(8), 591–598.

Ferrell, B. A., Stein, W. M., & Beck, J. C. (2000). The Geriatric Pain Measure: Validity, reliability, and factor analysis. *Journal of the American Geriatrics Society, 48*, 1669–1673.

Fisher, S. E., Burgio, L. D., Thorn, B. E., & Hardin, J. M. (2006). Obtaining self-report data from cognitively impaired elders: Methodological issues and clinical implications for nursing home pain assessment. *The Gerontologist, 46*(1), 81–88.

Fulmer, T., Mion, L. C., & Bottrell, M. M. (1996). Pain management protocol: NICHE faculty. *Geriatric Nursing, 17*, 222–226.

Gagliese, L., & Melzack, R. (1997). Chronic pain in elderly people. *Pain, 70*(1), 3–14.

Herr, K. (2004). Neuropathic pain: A guide to comprehensive assessment. *Pain Management Nursing, 5*(4 Suppl. 1), 9–18.

Herr, K. A., & Mobily, P. R. (1993). Comparison of selected pain assessment tools for use with the elderly. *Applied Nursing Research, 6*, 39–46.

Herr, K., Bjoro, K., & Decker, S. (2006). Tools for assessment of pain in nonverbal older adults with dementia: A state-of-the-science review. *Journal of Pain Symptom Management, 31*(2), 170–192.

Herr, K., Spratt, K., Mobily, P. A., & Richardson, G. (2004). Pain intensity assessment in older adults: Use of experimental pain to compare psychometric properties and usability of selected pain scales with younger adults. *Clinical Journal of Pain, 20*(4), 207–219.

Herr, K., Coyne, P. J., Key, T., Manworren, R., McCaffery, M., Merkel, S., et al. (2006). Pain assessment in the nonverbal patient: Position statement with clinical practice recommendations. *Pain Management Nursing, 7*(2), 44–52.

Hølen, J. C., Saltvedt, I., Fayers, P. M., Bjørnnes, M., Stenseth, G., Hval, B., et al. (2005). The Norwegian Doloplus-2, a tool for behavioural pain assessment: Translation and pilot-validation in nursing home patients with cognitive impairment. *Palliative Medicine, 19*(5), 411–417.

Horgas, A. L., & Dunn, K. (2001). Pain in nursing home residents: Comparison of residents' self report and nursing assistants' perceptions. *Journal of Gerontological Nursing, 27*, 44–53.

Hurley, A. C., Volicer, B. J., Hanrahan, P. A., Houde, S., & Volicer, L. (1992). Assessment of discomfort in advanced Alzheimer's patients. *Research in Nursing & Health, 15*(5), 369–377.

Joint Commission on Accreditation of Health Care Organizations (JCAHO). (2006). *Setting the standard: The joint commission and health care safety and quality.* Oakbrook Terrace, IL: Author.

Jones, K. R., Fink, R., Hutt, E., Vojir, C., Pepper, G. A., & Scott-Cawiezell, J. (2005). Measuring pain intensity in nursing home residents. *Journal of Pain Symptom Management, 30*(6), 519–527.

Kaasalainen, S., & Crook, J. (2004). An exploration of seniors' ability to report pain. *Clinical Nursing Research, 13*(3), 199–215.

Kim, E. J., & Buschmann, M. T. (2006). Reliability and validity of the Faces Pain Scale with older adults. *International Journal of Nursing Studies, 43*(4), 447–456.

Kovach, C., Noonan, P. E., Griffie, J., Muchka, S., & Weissman, D. E. (1999). Use of the assessment of discomfort in dementia protocol. *Applied Nursing Research, 14*(4), 193–200.

Kovach, C. R., Weissman, D. E., Griffie, J., Matson, S., & Muchka, S. (1999). Assessment and treatment of discomfort for people with late-stage dementia. *Journal Pain Symptom Management, 18*(6), 412–419.

Krause, S. J., & Backonja, M. (2003). Development of a neuropathic pain questionnaire. *Clinical Journal of Pain, 19,* 306–314.

Krulewitch, H., London, M. R., Skakel, V. J., Lundstedt, G. J., Thomason, H., & Brummel-Smith, K. (2000). Assessment of pain in cognitively impaired older adults: A comparison of pain assessment tools and their use by nonprofessional caregivers. *Journal of the American Geriatrics Society, 48*(12), 1607–1611.

Manworren, R. C., & Hynan, L. S. (2003). Clinical validation of FLACC: Preverbal patient pain scale. *Pediatric Nursing, 29*(2), 140–146.

McCaffery, M., & Pasero, C. (1999). *Pain clinical manual.* St Louis, MO: Mosby.

Meenan, R. F., Gertman, P. M., & Mason, J. H. (1980). Measuring health status in arthritis: The Arthritis Impact Measurement Scale. *Arthritis & Rheumatism (Arthritis Care & Research), 23,* 146–152.

Melzack, R. (1975). The McGill pain questionnaire: Major properties and scoring methods. *Pain, 1,* 277–299.

Miller, J., Neelon, V., Dalton, J., Ng'andu, N., Bailey, D. Jr., Layman, E., et al. (1996). The assessment of discomfort in elderly confused patients: a preliminary study. *Journal of Neuroscience Nursing, 28,* 175–182.

Morrison, R. S., Ahronheim, J. C., Morrison, G. R., Darling, E., Baskin, S. A., Morris, J., et al. (1998). Pain and discomfort associated with common hospital procedures and experiences. *Journal of Pain and Symptom Management, 15*(2), 91–101.

Mosier, R., Nusser-Gurlach, B., Manz, B., & Bergstrom, N. (1998, March). *Pain assessment in cognitively impaired and non-impaired elderly.* Presented at the 22nd Annual Midwest Nursing Research Society, Columbus, OH.

Nygaard H., & Jarland, M. (2006) The Checklist of Nonverbal Pain Indicators (CNPI): Testing of reliability and validity in Norwegian nursing homes. *Age and Ageing, 35*(1), 79–81.

Pautex, S., Harrmann, F., LeLous, P., Fabjan, M., Michel, J. P., & Gold, G. (2005). Feasibility and reliability of four pain self-assessment scales and correlation with an observational rating scale in hospitalized elderly demented patients. *Journals of Gerontology, Series Biol Sciences and Medical Sciences, 60*(4), 524–529.

Ren, X., Kazis, L., & Meenan, R. F. (1999). Short-form arthritis impact measurement scales 2: Tests of reliability and validity among patients with osteoarthritis. *Arthritis Care & Research, 12*(3), 163–171.

Scherder, E. J., & Bouma, A. (2000). Visual analogue scales for pain assessment in Alzheimer's disease. *Gerontology, 46*(1), 47–53.

Scherder, E., & van Manen, F. (2005). Pain in Alzheimer's disease: Nursing assistants' and patients' evaluations. *Journal of Advanced Nursing, 52*(2), 151–158.

Scherder, E., Bouma, A., Slaets, J., Ooms, M., Ribbe, M., Blok, A., et al. (2001). Repeated pain assessment in Alzheimer's disease. *Demenia and Geriatric Cognitive Disorders, 12*(6), 400–407.

Snow, A. L., Weber, J. B., O'Malley, K. J., Cody, M., Beck, C., Bruera, E., et al. (2004). NOPPAIN: A nursing assistant-administered pain assessment instrument for use in dementia. *Dementia and Geriatric Cognitive Disorders, 17*(3), 240–246.

Stuppy, D. J. (1998). The Faces Pain Scale: Reliability and validity with mature adults. *Applied Nursing Research, 11*(2), 84–89.

Taylor, L. J., & Herr, K. (2003). Pain intensity assessment: A comparison of selected pain intensity scales for use in cognitively intact and cognitively impaired African American older adults. *Pain Management Nursing, 4*(2), 87–95.

Taylor, L. J., Harris, J., Epps, C. D., & Herr, K. (2005). Psychometric evaluation of selected pain intensity scales for use with cognitively impaired and cognitively intact older adults. *Rehabilitation Nursing, 30*(2), 55–61.

Tsai, P. F., & Tak, S. (2003). Disease specific pain measures for osteoarthritis of the knee or hip. *Geriatric Nursing, 24*(2), 106–109.

U.S. Department of Health and Human Services. (2005). *Progress report on Alzheimer's disease.* NIH Publication No. 05–5724, Rockville, MD.

Warden, V., Hurley, A., & Volicer, L. (2003). Development and psychometric evaluation of the Pain Assessment in Advanced Dementia (PAINAD) scale. *Journal of the American Medical Directors Association, 4*(1), 9–15.

Ware, L. J., Epps, C. D., Herr, K., & Packard, A.(2006). Evaluation of the Revised Faces Pain Scale, Verbal Descriptor Scale, Numeric Rating Scale, and Iowa Pain Thermometer in older minority adults. *Pain Management Nursing, 7*(3), 117–125.

Wary, B., & Doloplus, C. (1999). Doloplus-2, a scale for pain measurement. (French) *Soins Gerontologie, 19,* 25–27.

Weiner, D. K., Peterson, B., & Keefe, E. J. (1999). Chronic pain-associated behaviors in the nursing home: Resident versus caregiver perceptions. *Pain, 80,* 577–588.

Weiner, D. K., Ladd, K. E., Pieper, C. F., & Keefe, F. J. (1995). Pain in the nursing home: Resident versus staff perceptions. *Journal of the American Geriatrics Society, 43*, SA2.

Wynne, C. F., Ling, S. M., & Remsburg, R. (2000). Comparison of pain assessment instruments in cognitively intact and cognitively impaired nursing home residents. *Geriatric Nursing, 21*(1), 20–23.

Zwakhalen, S., Hamers, J. P., & Berger, M. P. (2006). The psychometric quality and clinical usefulness of three pain assessment tools for elderly people with dementia. *Pain, 126*(1–3), 210–220.

Zwakhalen, S., Hamers, J. P., Abu-Saad, H. H., & Berger, M. (2006). Pain in elderly people with severe dementia: A systematic review of behavioural pain assessment tools. *BMC Geriatrics, 27*(6), 3.

CHAPTER 4

Pain Behaviors in the Older Adult

Melissa M. Tomesh

$\mathbf{P}$ain is a complex physiologic and emotional response. It is highly subjective and can only be defined by the person experiencing it. Chapter 3 discussed the importance of pain assessment in the treatment of pain in older adults. It also examined many of the pain assessment tools that can be used to help assess pain in the older adult, including those that can be used in cognitively impaired, nonverbal older adults. These tools rely heavily on pain behaviors in the assessment of pain. This chapter will define and provide examples of the different types of pain behaviors, as well as discuss the influence of pain beliefs and family/caregivers on pain behaviors.

PAIN BEHAVIORS

Pain behaviors are overt behaviors that communicate pain to others (Druley, Stephens, Martire, Ennis, & Wojno, 2003; Williamson, Robinson, & Melamed, 1997). Acute pain behaviors are fairly well recognized by health care providers and include behaviors such as grimacing, increased heart rate and blood pressure, perspiring, bracing the area of acute pain, and restricted movement. Persistent pain behaviors go beyond the autonomic signs of acute pain and are often ignored or not recognized as a significant aspect of pain assessment.

Persistent pain behaviors include verbal and nonverbal indicators of pain. Verbal complaints of pain may include moaning, groaning, and sighing.

Nonverbal displays of pain include overt displays of behavior, emotional upset, functional limitations, or use of pain-relieving aids. Overt displays of suffering include rubbing painful areas or facial expressions (such as wincing or clenching teeth). Emotional upset includes crying or irritability. Displays of functional limitations include such behaviors as slow, restricted movements, use of wheelchairs or assistive devices, or inactivity. Use of pain-relieving aids includes behaviors such as visits to health care providers, taking medications for pain, or using nonpharamacologic treatments. Pain-related behaviors are an important aspect of assessment, because they provide additional and functional information related to the patient's pain. It is noted however, that pain-related behaviors can be exaggerated or maladaptive and need to be accurately assessed. Table 4.1 lists the types of pain behaviors and provides examples of clinical manifestations.

Each individual has a set of pain beliefs, or attitudes and feelings about pain, that affect that individual's response to pain. When assessing pain in the older adult, it is important to remember that these beliefs may influence not only their display of pain behaviors but also their perception of pain. These beliefs can become barriers to accurate assessment and treatment of pain. Some common beliefs in the older population include regarding pain as a normal part of growing old, fearing the need for tests or medications that have side effects or high costs associated with them, or fearing addiction to strong

TABLE 4.1   Types of Pain Behaviors

Verbalizations/ Vocalizations	Overt Displays of Suffering	Emotional Upset	Displays of Functional Limitations	Use of Pain-Relieving Aids
Verbal complaints of pain	Rubbing joints	Crying	Stiff, slow, restricted movement	Medications
Moaning, groaning	Facial expressions (such as grimacing, wincing, clenching teeth)	Irritability		Visits to health care providers
Sighing		Agitation	Use of supports (bracing oneself)	Use of ice packs or heating pads
	Restless body movements		Use of wheelchairs	
	Sitting in a semi-recumbent position with one leg extended		Assistive devices	
			Limping	
			Inactivity	

analgesics (Jones, Fink, Hutt, Vojir, Pepper, et al., 2005; Miaskowski, 2000; Stolee, Hillier, Esbaugh, Bol, McKellar, et al., 2005).

Older adults living in nursing homes and/or who have caregivers have additional barriers to accurate assessment of pain. Elderly persons with caregivers might fear being labeled a "bad patient" or a "complainer." Many nursing home residents may not have the will or capacity to complain of pain (Weiner & Rudy, 2002). Behaviors such as aggression, resistance, and irritability may be due to pain, but are often attributed to conditions such as dementia (Stolee et al., 2005). Due to the high incidence in pain in nursing homes, pain behaviors may be overlooked by some caregivers because they occur so often (Weiner & Rudy, 2002). Patients newly admitted to nursing homes are a challenge for caregivers to assess, because their baseline behavior is unknown. Mentes, Teer, and Cadogan (2004) suggest scheduling a family interview on admission to a nursing home to discuss the relative's pain expression and personal history.

Caregivers need to be aware of pain behaviors and incorporate them in their assessment of pain. It is noted, however, that self-report should always be the first approach to assessing pain, when possible. Observable pain behaviors are not always present even in the presence of pain (Jones et al., 2005). Older individuals may have physical limitations that do not allow them to express certain pain behaviors, such as paralysis or blunted facial expressions, as in a patient with Parkinson's Disease (Kaasalainen & Crook, 2003).

Assessment of pain-related behaviors may be the only indication of pain in a cognitively impaired older adult. Chapter 3 discusses several valid tools for assessing pain in cognitively impaired older adults that include nonverbal pain-related behaviors.

INFLUENCE OF FAMILY MEMBERS

Assessment and knowledge of pain behaviors is equally important for non-cognitively impaired older adults and families. Pain is highly subjective, and pain behaviors can be influenced by interactions with family members. Solicitous behavior by spouses, such as expressions of concern or support and provision of assistance related to the patient's pain are thought to be reinforcing for subsequent pain behaviors (Romano, Turner, Friedman, Bulcroft, Jensen, et al., 1992). In a study of 50 chronic pain patients, Romano and colleagues (1995) found that spouses' solicitous responses were related to physical disability and increased frequency in pain behaviors. A study of 52 patients with rheumatoid arthritis (Williamson, Robinson, & Melamed, 1997) demonstrated that pain behaviors occurred more frequently in the presence of the spouse than in the presence of a neutral observer.

A spouse's response to pain behaviors can influence the older chronic pain patient's level of pain as well as level of activity. In a study of 32 chronic pain patients and their spouses, Flor, Kerns, and Turk (1987) found that positive reinforcement of pain behaviors was related to increased pain levels in patients. The same study found that patients with spouses who minimized the patient's pain had higher levels of activity. Solicitous behaviors tend to encourage the sick role by discouraging activity, which can lead to greater disability (Romano, Jensen, Turner, Good, & Hops, 2000). Figure 4.1 displays how these reinforcing consequences and solicitous behaviors can lead to increased pain and pain behaviors, lower levels of activity, and increased disability.

It is vital that a maladaptive pain behavior cycle be recognized and corrected. If allowed to continue, it can have serious consequences for the individual as well as the family. Individual consequences of this vicious cycle include loss of functional abilities, depression, anxiety, and problems with social

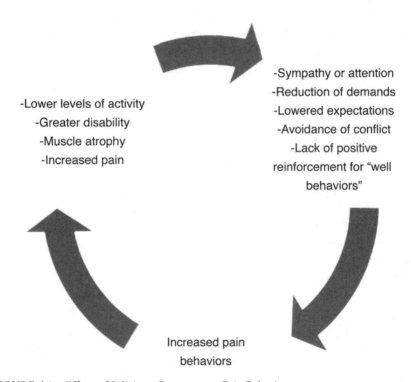

-Sympathy or attention
-Reduction of demands
-Lowered expectations
-Avoidance of conflict
-Lack of positive reinforcement for "well behaviors"

-Lower levels of activity
-Greater disability
-Muscle atrophy
-Increased pain

Increased pain behaviors

FIGURE 4.1   Effects of Solicitous Responses on Pain Behaviors

interaction (Chandra & Ozturk, 2005). Spouses of chronic pain patients can also suffer physical and emotional consequences of pain behaviors if a maladaptive cycle persists. Flor, Turk, and Scholz (1987) discovered that 86% of the spouses of chronic pain patients experienced pain symptoms at least once a week. In a study of 101 women with osteoarthritis and their husbands, Druley and colleagues (2003) found that wives who demonstrated high levels of pain behaviors and depressive symptoms had husbands who had increased depressive symptoms and anger. On the other hand, husbands who had wives who had depressive symptoms but did not demonstrate high levels of pain behavior did not show in increase in depression or anger.

Adaptive Behaviors

It is possible to break the maladaptive pain behavior cycle and remain supportive. Teaching family members and/or caregivers to promote adaptive or positive behaviors is crucial in changing the behaviors that facilitate the maladaptive cycle. Facilitative comments such as: "I know you can do it" instead of solicitous comments like "I'll do that" can reinforce "well behaviors." Redirecting support and expressions of concern to "well behaviors" can minimize the reinforcement of the "sick role." Encouraging older adults suffering from persistent pain to keep a diary of daily activities, and slowly increasing the amount of exercise and activity can help emphasize the importance of the return of function. Encouraging the family and/or caregivers to increase social activities can help to prevent social isolation and improve social interactions. For example, an older person with chronic or persistent pain may not want to participate in any social activities because it may precipitate an exacerbation of their pain. A family member can acknowledge this concern but modify the activity, such as playing bridge for one hour rather than two or three hours. This action by the family member promotes social interaction, yet acknowledges the older person's concern.

The following case study further demonstrates strategies that can be used to promote pain management in an older adult.

Case Study

Marge is a 73-year-old developmentally disabled woman who lives in a group home. She is able to communicate, but she is considerably cognitively impaired. Her niece, Shelly, is her legal guardian. Shelly lives in a nearby city but has a family of her own to care for. Shelly became legal guardian when her father, Marge's brother, died of a heart attack several years ago. Shelly cares very deeply for Marge and visits often. She takes time off of work to take Marge to medical appointments when she can but trusts the caregivers at the group home to take care of Marge. The group home and caregivers have been Marge's home and family since Marge's mother died 16 years ago.

Recently Marge has been complaining more frequently of back pain. She has had chronic back pain for several years due to arthritis but has been more vocal about the pain recently. Her primary physician gave her narcotic medications for the pain and referred her to a pain clinic for further evaluation. A series of lumbar epidural injections was trialed, but was not beneficial for Marge. She is seen by a nurse practitioner in the pain clinic for medication management of her persistent pain. Shelly accompanies Marge to her appointment and voices concerns about Marge not receiving adequate pain medication. Shelly becomes tearful and states that she has tried to talk with the caregivers, but they seem to think that Marge doesn't always need strong pain medications. They have voiced concerns about the side effects and fears of addiction to Shelly and they feel they know what is best for Marge.

The nurse practitioner suggests a care meeting with the caregivers, Shelly, Marge, and herself to discuss Marge's pain management. Shelly agrees with this plan and an appointment is set. The nurse practitioner starts the meeting by asking Marge about her pain. Marge states "my back hurts" and states that her pain is an eight on a scale of 0 to 10 but is unable to give any more details about the nature of her pain. The nurse practitioner asks the caregivers how they assess Marge's pain. Many examples are given from the caregivers, including observation of pain behaviors (specifically facial expressions, asking for pain pills, and inactivity), simply asking if pain is present, and monitoring Marge's mood and sleep pattern. The nurse practitioner commends them on their multiple ways of assessing Marge's pain and their individualized approach.

The nurse practitioner asks Marge what seems to help her back the most. Marge answers that her pain pills and lying down help the most. The nurse practitioner then asks the caregivers what they most often do for Marge's pain. The caregivers state that they often try a mild analgesic, like acetaminophen, first. When that does not help, they will try to distract her with an activity, have her lie down, or try an ice pack. They will give a stronger pain medication from time to time. They think the stronger pain medications are helpful but worry about side effects; therefore, they are reluctant to give them to her. The nurse practitioner reviews side effects with the caregivers and encourages them to contact her if they notice any side effects. She also commends them on their various pain management strategies but encourages them to try the stronger pain medication on a regular basis, rather than a last resort for severe pain.

The nurse practitioner discusses goals for pain management with Marge, the caregivers, and Shelly. Shelly states that she feels better after this meeting about how the caregivers are assessing Marge's pain, but she would like the caregivers to be a little more proactive with the treatment of pain. Shelly states that when she comes to visit, Marge is lying down and seems to be in pain when she sits up to visit with Shelly. The caregivers would also like Marge to be able to be more active and be able to change positions without so much pain. Marge would like to be able to do her share of the work around the group home. They are willing to try giving the medications on a regular schedule. They agree that if side effects become a problem they will contact the nurse practitioner and they can trial other medications.

At a follow-up visit one month later, Marge continues to rate her pain as an 8 on a scale of 0–10 but reports her pain as much improved. She states that she is able to perform all her household chores and only needs a short rest in the afternoon. Shelly reports that Marge is more willing to go on short social excursions and has less verbal complaints of pain. A written note by the caregivers of the group home also report fewer observable pain-related behaviors.

SUMMARY

Pain behaviors can provide valuable information on the nature and function of persistent pain in older adults. It is important to include assessment of verbal and nonverbal pain behaviors. It is also important to assess family members for solicitous behaviors and provide corrective measures to avoid maladaptive cycles of chronic pain.

REFERENCES

Chandra, A., & Ozturk, A. (2005). Quality of life issues and assessment tools as they relate to patients with chronic nonmalignant pain. *Hospital Topics Sarasota, 83,* 33–37.

Druley, J. A., Stephens, M. P., Martire, L. M., Ennis, N., & Wojno, W. (2003). Emotional congruence in older couples coping with wives' osteoarthritis: Exacerbating effects of pain behavior. *Psychology and Aging, 18,* 406–414.

Flor, H., Kerns, R. D., & Turk, D. C. (1987). The role of spouse reinforcement, perceived pain, and activity levels of chronic pain patients. *Journal of Psychosomatic Research, 31,* 251–259.

Flor, H., Turk, D. C., & Scholz, O. B. (1987). Impact of chronic pain on the spouse: Marital, emotional and physical consequences. *Journal of Psychosomatic Research, 31,* 63–71.

Jones, K. R., Fink, R., Hutt, E., Vojir, C., Pepper, G., Scott-Cawiezell, J., et al. (2005). Measuring pain intensity in nursing home residents. *Journal of Pain and Symptom Management, 30,* 519–527.

Kaasalainen, S., & Crook, J. (2003). A comparison of pain-assessment tools for use with elderly long-term-care residents. *Canadian Journal of Nursing Research, 35,* 58–71.

Mentes, J. C., Teer, J., & Cadogan, M. P. (2004). The pain experience of cognitively impaired nursing home residents: Perceptions of family members and certified nursing assistants. *Pain Management Nursing, 5,* 118–125.

Miaskowski, C. (2000). The impact of age on a patient's perception of pain and ways it can be managed. *Pain Management Nursing, 1,* 2–7.

Romano, J. M., Jensen, M. P., Turner, J. A., Good, A. B., & Hops, H. (2000). Chronic pain patient-partner interactions: Further support for a behavioral model of chronic pain. *Behavior Therapy, 31,* 415–440.

Romano, J. M., Turner, J. A., Friedman, L. S., Bulcroft, R. A., Jensen, M. P., Hops, H., et al. (1992). Sequential analysis of chronic pain behaviors and spouse responses. *Journal of Consulting and Clinical Psychology, 60,* 777–782.

Romano, J. M., Turner, J. A., Jensen, M. P., Friedman, L. S., Bulcroft, R. A., Hops, H., et al. (1995). Chronic pain patient-spouse behavioral interactions predict patient disability. *Pain, 63,* 353–360.

Stolee, P., Hillier, L. M., Esbaugh, J., Bol, N., McKellar, L., & Gauthier, N. (2005). Instruments for the assessment of pain in older persons with cognitive impairment. *Journal of the American Geriatrics Society, 53,* 319–326.

Weiner, D. K., & Rudy, T. E. (2002). Attitudinal barriers to effective treatment of persistent pain in nursing home residents. *Journal of the American Geriatrics Society, 50,* 2035–2040.

Williamson, D., Robinson, M. E., & Melamed, B. (1997). Pain behavior, spouse responsiveness, and marital satisfaction in patients with rheumatoid arthritis. *Behavior Modification, 21,* 97–118.

CHAPTER 5

Relationship of Pain and Sleep in Older Adults

Kerri M. Crank

Pain is a major health problem worldwide that affects quality of life, mood, and sleep, leading to tremendous economic and personal costs (Smith & Haythornthwaite, 2003). The effects of pain on mood and quality of life, combined with both pathological sleep problems and the normal changes of aging, further influence costs in the elderly. The lack of knowledge of health care providers in sleep assessment leads to untreated sleep problems that can affect pain perception as well. This chapter will review normal sleep and changes related to aging; sleep disorders common in the elderly; and the relationships between pain, sleep, and depression. Clinical implications and potential treatment options will also be presented.

NORMAL SLEEP

Sleep is an active process regulated by behavioral, neuroendocrine, and central nervous system factors. Carskadon and Dement (2000) define sleep as "a reversible behavioral state of perceptual disengagement from and unresponsiveness to the environment" (p.15). Sleep is divided into two stages, non-rapid eye movement (NREM) and rapid eye movement (REM) sleep. NREM sleep is subdivided into four stages, best noted during an electroencephalogram (EEG), characterized by progressively slowing brain waves. The four stages of sleep parallel a continuum of arousal threshold from low in stage 1 to high in stage 4. Stages 3 and 4 are typically referred to as slow wave sleep (SWS) or deep sleep. NREM has been described as a quiet brain in an active body, whereas REM sleep is described as an active brain in a paralyzed body. REM sleep is commonly referred to as dreaming sleep and is characterized by periods of activity with episodes of quiescence noted on the EEG. Observable signs of REM sleep include rapid eye movement, twitching muscles, and irregular breathing patterns, alternating with periods of stillness.

Adults generally begin a sleep cycle in NREM sleep. Progression is seen through the various stages of NREM sleep. First onset of REM sleep is typically 80 minutes after sleep onset. A sleep cycle is typically completed in 90 minutes, with the average adult going through five cycles per night. A typical sleep cycle is illustrated in Figure 5.1.

Sleep cycles are consistent in content, but the amount of time spent in each stage varies throughout the night. The combination and distribution of sleep cycles throughout the night are referred to as sleep architecture (Carskadon & Dement, 2000). NREM sleep represents about 75% to 80% of total sleep time, with approximately 50% spent in stage 2 sleep. Slow wave sleep comprises 13% to 23% of total sleep time and is most prevalent during the first third of the total sleep time. REM sleep dominates the last third of sleep and is generally 20% to 25% of total sleep time. REM sleep is correlated with temperature changes driven by circadian rhythms. There are several factors that can affect the quality of sleep and sleep architecture.

Quality of sleep is related to many factors, including the aging process, changes in circadian rhythms, temperature extremes, drugs, sleep disorders, medical or psychiatric disorders, and pain. The preceding factors can change

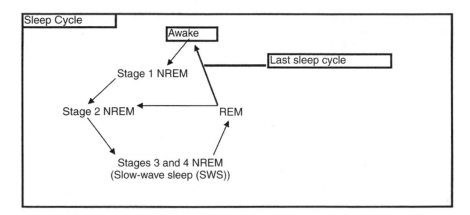

FIGURE 5.1   Typical Sleep Cycle

sleep architecture and can cause the perception of poor sleep. Circadian rhythm shifts occur with travel across time zones and with shift work, leading to changes in sleep onset and the distribution of the various sleep stages during sleep time (Carskadon & Dement, 2000). REM sleep, which is particularly temperature sensitive, is often disrupted by temperature extremes but is also light-dark sensitive (Cagnacci, Elliott, & Yen, 1992; Carskadon & Dement, 2000; McGinty & Szymusiak, 1990). Part of temperature sensitivity may be related to the inability to thermoregulate during REM sleep.

Drugs can have a potent effect on sleep (Carskadon & Dement, 2000). REM sleep and SWS have been shown to be suppressed with the use of benzodiazepines (Carskadon & Dement, 2000), opiates (Cronin, Keifter, Davies, King, & Bixler, 2001), and tetrahydrocanabinol (THC) (Carskadon & Dement, 2000). REM sleep is suppressed by antidepressants (tricyclics, selective serotonin reuptake inhibitors, and MAOI). Alcohol ingestion within a couple of hours of bedtime can result in initially suppressed REM sleep with a rebound of REM sleep noted later in the sleep cycle. Sleep disorders, medical diseases, and psychiatric problems can cause disruptions in sleep architecture, a decrease in total sleep time, and perceived poor sleep quality.

Effects of Aging on Sleep

Aging is responsible for many changes in sleep. Infants enter sleep through REM sleep with NREM/REM sleep cycles occurring every 50–60 minutes (Carskadon & Dement, 2000). NREM sleep staging is poorly differentiated at birth, developing during the first two to six months. Sleep is stable in early childhood, with significant SWS most notable. Important changes occur at puberty in sleep architecture, including increased total sleep time, decreased SWS, and a shift in circadian rhythms. Decreased SWS leads to a decrease in arousal threshold and more nighttime awakenings. Also occurring at this time is a shift in circadian rhythms that leads to a delay in sleep onset and later morning wakening. Combining this shift in sleep times with an increased need for sleep can lead to a sleep deficit and increased daytime sleepiness. This shift will gradually change during the third decade of life. Sleep will remain relatively stable through middle age with the exception of SWS, which continues to decline (Buysse, Browman, Monk, Reynolds, Fasiczka, et al., 1992).

There are sleep changes that are unique in the older adult (Ganguli, Reynolds, & Gilby, 1996). Controversy exists in defining what normal sleep is in the elderly because of the likelihood of contributing factors including pain, medical problems, and the aging of other organ systems that can affect sleep, such as nocturia in the male with an enlarged prostrate, or the female entering

TABLE 5.1   Sleep Hygiene Measures

Sleep Hygiene Measures
Keep consistent sleep and wake times.
Keep bed time to within 30 minutes of sleep time.
Avoid napping or keep to less than 20 minutes.
Exercise regularly, 30–40 minutes per day.
Get 1/2 hour of bright light in the morning hours.
If awake during the night, avoid bright light.
Bathe in the evening within 2 hours of bed.
Avoid caffeine, alcohol, and nicotine within six hours of bedtime.
Avoid recreational drugs.
Eat a light snack before bed if necessary.
Establish a bedtime routine that is distinctly different from daytime routines.
Keep bedroom comfortable in temperature, darkness, and sound.
Set aside worry time.
Avoid the bedroom for anything besides sleep and sexual activity.

menopause who is experiencing night sweats (Bliwise, 2000). Occasionally, sleep problems may be related to psychosocial factors like the loss of a spouse or retirement. Sleep disturbances may be caused by the lack or loss of good sleep hygiene measures as outline in Table 5.1.

Along with these potential causes of sleep disturbance, there are definite changes in sleep noted on polysomnography in older adults. Some changes include decreased sleep efficiency and diminished SWS. Sleep efficiency in older adults is typically around 85% compared to 90%–95% in younger adults (Bliwise, 2000). In addition, there is a decrease in SWS and, in some men by age 60, no SWS (Bliwise, 2000). This can lead to lighter sleep, with more frequent arousals, and less total sleep time. Added to this are circadian changes related to temperature and the endocrine system that cause a shift in normal sleep times, generally toward earlier sleep and waking patterns. Some of the circadian changes may be related to social factors that weaken "zeitgebers" or cues that let your body know when it is time to sleep. These include consistent wake and bedtimes, bedtime routines, consistent scheduling of activities, and the amount of bright light exposure in the morning (Bliwise, 2000; Campbell & Zulley, 1989; McGinty & Szymusiak, 1990; Monk, Buysse, Carrier, Billy, & Rose, 2001; Myers & Badia, 1995; Naylor,

Penev, Orbeta, Janssen, Ortiz, et al., 2000). Even if these factors do not change total sleep time, they may cause the perception of poorer sleep quality.

SLEEP DISORDERS IN OLDER ADULTS

While changes in sleep patterns influence sleep in the elderly, it is not the only cause of sleep problems. There are sleep disorders that affect the elderly just as in young adults. Prevalence of these disorders increasing with age is controversial, with recent studies demonstrating conflicting results. Noteworthy sleep disorders include insomnia, sleep apnea, and periodic limb movements.

Insomnia

There is some disagreement whether older adults suffer from insomnia more often than younger adults, partially because of the known decrease in sleep efficiency defined as normal in the elderly. Insomnia can also be related to each individual's perception of sleep. The following example can illustrate this difference in perception. Two individuals may have a total sleep time of 6 hours. One sleeps soundly for 6 straight hours, waking rested. The other falls asleep at 9 P.M., is awake for two hours during the night, then falls back to sleep, waking feeling rested at 5 A.M. Both have the same amount of total sleep time, but one may perceive insomnia where the other does not.

Another factor predisposing the older adult to insomnia includes increased NREM stage 1 sleep (lighter sleep) with less SWS and early morning awakening as a result of changing circadian patterns that lead to more time awake in bed (Bliwise, 2000; Myers & Badia, 1995; Naylor et al., 2000). Behaviors that reinforce sleeplessness then can perpetuate and worsen insomnia, such as poor bedtime routines, excessive daytime napping, staying in bed when not asleep, and scheduling inconsistencies (Campbell & Zulley, 1989; Myers & Badia, 1995). In addition, people with disrupted sleep due to sleep apnea can appear to experience insomnia, leading to misdiagnosis and erroneous treatment (Foley, Monjan, Brown, Simonsick, Wallace, et al., 1995).

Sleep Apnea

Sleep apnea is a relatively common disorder throughout the life span, particularly in men. Estrogen production in childbearing females provides protection from sleep apnea initially, and, while the difference between genders fades with the onset of menopause, sleep apnea continues to be more prevalent in

TABLE 5.2   Risk Factors Related to Sleep Apnea in the Elderly

Risk Factors of Sleep Apnea in the Elderly	
Increased body weight	Diminished muscle endurance
Diminished lung capacity	Diminished thyroid function
Decreased ventilatory control	Increased sleep fragmentation
Increased upper airway collapsibility	Decreased slow-wave sleep

men. It is hypothesized that sleep apnea is age-dependent, occurring more frequently in the elderly than younger adults (Bliwise, 2000). Preliminary data support this, but further evidence is needed to confirm these findings. Several risk factors predispose older adults to sleep apnea and are outlined in Table 5.2. The outcomes of untreated sleep apnea include increased mortality; neurobehavioral morbidity including "sleep attacks;" memory difficulties and ischemic events; cardiovascular morbidity including hypertension, myocardial infarction, or ischemia; arrhythmias; and other end organ damage such as renal failure (Bedard, Montplaisir, Richer, Roulou, & Malo, 1991).

Periodic Limb Movements (PLM)

Periodic limb movement (PLM) is another disorder of sleep. The impact of PLMs on morbidity in the elderly is unknown at this time. An age-dependent increased incidence of PLMs has been noted, but its significance is questionable, as its presence does not necessarily mean sleep disturbance (Bliwise, 2000; Hirshkowitz, Moore, Hamilton, Rando, & Karacan, 1992). PLM can be caused by a deficit or derangement in transmission of dopamine in the basal ganglia, lumbosacral narrowing due to osteoarthritic changes and disc abnormalities in the spine, venous insufficiency, high normal or elevated blood urea nitrogen (BUN) levels, sleep apnea, and anemia, all of which are more prevalent in older people. When associated with restless legs syndrome or pain, PLMs become more clinically significant due to the resulting disruption in sleep and increase in daytime sleepiness. Lobbezoo and colleagues (2003) examined individuals with cervicospinal and craniomandibular pain and noted that subjects with higher pain scores and more areas of pain suffered more from PLM and restless legs. In addition, more impairment was found in those older than 55, but the number was not statistically significant.

These sleep disorders, along with the changes that naturally occur in sleep, result in disrupted sleep and drowsiness that, left untreated, lead to decreased quality of life, diminished coping abilities, and increased mood instability. This can have a negative impact on pain and the treatment of pain.

RELATIONSHIP BETWEEN PAIN AND SLEEP

The interdependent relationship between pain and sleep is complex. Pain can cause difficulty with sleep onset and sleep maintenance (Aigner, Graf, Freidl, Prause, Weiss, et al., 2003). The treatment of pain with opioids diminishes REM and SWS percentages, leading to nonrestorative, disrupted sleep. Untreated or inadequately treated pain can lead to problems with depression and anxiety that cause additional sleep disruption. On the other hand, poor sleep contributes to increased mood instability and decreased coping ability, leading to increased perception of pain. Several studies demonstrate that nonrestorative sleep can cause pain, whereas good sleep can ameliorate the effects of pain. Depression also appears to be a factor in both pain and sleep, and its independent contributions will also be explored.

The Effect of Sleep on Pain

There currently is no conclusive evidence that disrupted sleep is an independent cause of persistent pain (Smith & Haythornthwaite, 2004). The limitations of current studies include a lack of polysomnographic evidence of sleep disruption. Several studies measure sleep only by questionnaire regarding perception of sleep. Despite this, there is evidence that sleep, while not an independent factor, contributes to the perception of pain.

Poor sleep may be related to many factors, including cognitive behavioral factors such as depression and anxiety, and sleep hygiene, more than to pain severity. Several studies discuss the relationship of poor sleep and sleep deprivation on pain. The possibility of sleep disruption and direct effects on the nociceptive pain process with subjects deprived of sleep was first noted in 1934 (Cooperman, Mullin, & Kleitman, 1934). Subjects were noted to experience a decrease in pain threshold that was restored with recovery sleep. Corroborating this, Onen and colleagues (2001) report that healthy males deprived of sleep for 40 hours experienced hyperalgesia to mechanical stimuli. This was reversed with the recovery of slow-wave sleep. Studies performed by Moldofsky and Scarisbrick (1976) more than 25 years ago demonstrated that individuals whose stage 4 NREM sleep was selectively disrupted led to complaints of "fibrositis," currently referred to as fibromyalgia. Moldofsky and Scarisbrick (1976) also noted that subjects who exercised regularly had less pain when SWS was disrupted, suggesting a possible protective value of regular exercise. Recent replications of these studies have demonstrated mixed results but generally suggest a relationship between diminished SWS and pain sensitivity (Lentz, Landis, Rothermel, & Shaver, 1999).

Poor sleep and sleep deprivation may be signs of insomnia and depression, both known to be a factor in perception of acute and persistent chronic pain. Koopman and colleagues (2002) observed that individuals who had difficulty falling asleep had greater pain levels and more symptoms of depression. Those individuals who woke during the night and those who had difficulty waking in the morning reported higher levels of depression, suggesting that pain and sleep are both affected by depression. Additional supporting evidence comes from a study of pain clinic patients in a metropolitan area. Patient self-reports of poor sleep were associated with more anxiety, depression, and irritability; higher levels of pain; more rest periods during the day; and more disability than those who reported good sleep (Pilowsky, Crettenden, & Townley, 1985).

The findings in these studies support that sleep alone and in combination with depression play a role in pain intensity and create a significant impact on people who experience pain. However, pain also affects sleep, causing many of the same sleep problems that cause pain.

The Effect of Pain on Sleep

Many of the same sleep problems that contribute to pain perception are caused by pain. Sleep disturbance is often caused by pain. Sleep disturbances include changes in slow-wave sleep (SWS), stage I and II NREM sleep, changes in total sleep time, prolonged sleep onset, and frequent sleep disruption. The type of pain appears to influences the sleep disturbance noted. There is also a difference between the effects of acute pain versus those of persistent pain.

Drewes and colleagues (1997) recognized that different sources of pain produce differing EEG patterns and changes in sleep. An increased alpha wave intrusion during slow-wave sleep was noted with introduction of slow onset muscle pain that was not noted with joint pain. Landis, Levine, and Robinson (1988) observed rats with and without chronic arthritis pain. Rats with chronic arthritis pain had a more than 50% reduction in SWS than rats without arthritis. Sleep deprivation further decreased pain threshold, and total sleep time was significantly reduced, with most difficulty noted in sleep maintenance. In a human study, people living with osteoarthritis experienced more impaired sleep with frequent awakening, prolonged time to sleep onset, more stage 1 NREM sleep, and less stage 2 NREM sleep, suggesting more sleep disruption (Wilcox, Brenes, Levine, Sevick, Shumaker, et al., 2000). In a related study of individuals who had total hip arthropathy, older adults (> 65 years) had better improvement in sleep after surgery, with a significant reduction in time spent in bed and more total sleep time, less limb movements and activity during sleep, and less disrupted sleep (Fielden, Gander, Horne, Lewer, Green, et al., 2003). Drewes and colleagues (2000) found that older individuals with rheumatoid arthritis who reported increased stiffness, increased pain, and increased disease activity encountered more insomnia, an increase in SWS, and decreased stage 2 sleep. This study supports the role of SWS as physically restorative, but further studies are needed to confirm this.

In studies of other sources of pain, Boeve and colleagues (2002) examined individuals after burn injuries. Burn pain was associated with insomnia, perceived poor sleep quality, and altered sleep patterns. The authors noted the potential impact of psychiatric problems on sleep in this group, particularly the possibility of post-traumatic stress. In a study of patients with spinal cord injury (SCI), subjects with SCI who experienced continuous pain had more impaired sleep by report, more anxiety, and higher pain intensity scores (Budh, Hulting, & Lundeberg, 2005).

Call-Schmidt and Richardson (2003) studied patients from an interdisciplinary outpatient pain clinic in Utah. They also found that patients with persistent pain had a high prevalence of sleep disturbance. Smith and Haythornthwaite (2004) noted that 50% of patients with chronic pain experienced sleep disturbance. The subjects reported frequent sleep fragmentation, longer times to sleep onset, and decreased quality of sleep.

Wittig and colleagues (1982) documented increased total sleep time in patients with chronic pain. The higher the level of pain, the more sleep problems were noted. The authors recognized that people with chronic pain frequently have depression that further affects sleep. It is also noted that pain behaviors may condition poor sleep, perpetuating the problem. Pain behaviors such as lying down in bed during the day to help alleviate pain, staying in bed while awake, loss of schedule consistency, and lack of bedtime routines that differ from daytime activities affect nighttime sleep. In addition, the medications used to alleviate pain, such as opioids, antidepressants, and hypnotics, negatively affected the sleep cycle, as do other nonpharmacologic comfort measures. For example, repositioning to find comfort from low back pain or neck pain results in more frequent nighttime awakening. Interestingly, older persons in this study actually had sounder sleep, potentially because of adaptation to chronic pain.

Sleep studies on animals as well as humans suggest that pain influences sleep. However, limitations of many of the studies on sleep and pain, including small sample sizes, inadequate sleep assessment, lack of pain variable control, and predominately white populations, demonstrate the need for more studies in this area.

The Role of Mood Disorders on Pain and Sleep

Several of the studies cited thus far have indicated that mood disorders, particularly depression, affect both sleep and pain (Budh, Hulting, & Lundeberg, 2005; Boeve, Aaron, Martin-Herz, Peterson, Cain, et al., 2002; Call-Schmidt & Richardson, 2003; Koopman, Nouriani, Erickson, Anupindi, Butler, et al., 2002; Lobbezoo, Visscher, & Naeije, 2003; Pilowsky, Crettenden, & Townley, 1985; Smith & Haythornthwaite, 2004; Wilcox et al., 2000). Koopman and colleagues (2002) observed that individuals who had problems falling asleep or woke during the night had higher levels of depression, as did those who had difficulty waking in the morning, thus suggesting that pain and sleep are both affected by depression. The interrelationship between depression, pain, and sleep is indeterminate and no causal relationships have been identified. The effects appear to be multidirectional among all factors. Figure 5.2 illustrates the multidirectional relationship among these factors.

Sleep deprivation is known to cause problems with mood, particularly depression (Borbely & Wirz-Justice, 1982; Dinges, Pack, Williams, Gillen, Powell, et al., 1997; Friedman, Globus, & Huntley, 1977; Pilcher & Huffcutt, 1996). Depression has clear effects on sleep, including interruptions in sleep maintenance, change in proportion of sleep, change in the pattern of sleep stages (less SWS), and changes within REM sleep (shorter duration to REM onset and duration of first REM episode). Density of REM sleep is increased in both first and total REM sleep time. Borbely and Wirz-Justice note that features typically seen in depression are also seen in the elderly, raising the

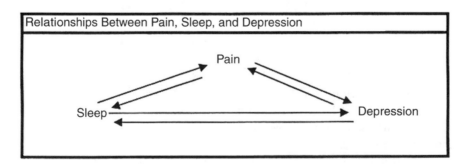

Relationships Between Pain, Sleep, and Depression

Pain

Sleep

Depression

FIGURE 5.2   Multidirectional Relationship between Depression, Pain, and Sleep

possibility of precocious aging. It is noted, however, that this study was conducted before the advent of SSRIs, which are known to actually decrease the total amount of REM sleep time and percentage of sleep.

Individuals experiencing pain have shorter total sleep times with more sleep disruption noted, resulting in a state of sleep deprivation. A meta-analysis on sleep deprivation demonstrated that partial sleep deprivation has a greater overall impact than short-term or long-term sleep deprivation, with the greatest effect on mood. "On average, sleep deprived subjects reported mood ratings that were over 3 standard deviations worse than those of non-sleep deprived subjects." (Pilcher & Huffcutt, 1996, p. 324). Borbely and Wirz-Justice (1982) noted clinical improvement correlated with an increased percentage of REM sleep in the later part of sleep, replicating normal sleep. Advanced sleep therapy was used to prolong the time to onset of REM sleep, and sleep latency was shortened. Long-term sleep complaints in persistent pain are more a result of mood disturbance. Insomnia develops as a secondary symptom of depression in some patients (Smith & Haythornthwaite, 2000). It is possible that behaviors used to cope with pain may actually perpetuate insomnia. Examples of these behaviors include decreased activity levels, increased napping, and pairing of the bedroom with pain rather than sleep.

Clinical Implications and Treatment

Pain, sleep, and depression are interrelated and influence the quality of life. The literature indicates that treatment of one disorder provides some relief, but a multidimensional approach can provide additional relief and improved quality of life. To achieve this goal, each disorder needs to be appropriately assessed and treated to achieve the best results on each individual's health. Moreover, there are special considerations that need to be addressed in the older adult.

Assessment

Proper treatment depends on accurate assessment. There are several tools for the measurement of depression, sleep, and pain. Pain assessment tools have been discussed in detail in Chapter 3. Sleep and depression rating tools also take pain into consideration. Sleep quality questionnaires include Leed's Sleep Evaluation Questionnaire, Pittsburgh Sleep Quality Index, Sleep Impairment Index, and St. Mary's Hospital Sleep Questionnaire. Sleep diaries include the National Sleep Foundation Sleep Diary, Pittsburgh Sleep Diary, and Sleep Log. Tools to measure daytime sleepiness include the Epworth

Sleepiness Scale, Functional Outcomes of Sleep Questionnaire, and the Stanford Sleepiness Scale. Rating scales for depression include the Patient Health Questionnaire (PHQ-9), Beck Depression Inventory, the Center for Epidemiological Studies Depression (CES-D) scale, and the Profile of Mood States (POMS).

The Pittsburgh Sleep Quality Index (PSQI) with the Pittsburgh Sleep Diary (PSD) render the most relevant clinical information. Both tools are easy to read and complete. The PSQI is quantifiable, making it an ideal tool for research. In addition, the Epworth Sleepiness Scale (ESS) is fast and easy to complete, an important feature in clinical practice. While many scales are not used in their exact form, the questions remain similar and provide relevant clinical data from which a diagnosis is made.

Treatment

Depression

Depression needs to be adequately treated to maximize treatment of pain and sleep disturbances. Counseling and antidepressants not only treat depression but also help improve sleep and pain. Counseling can aid in the development of coping strategies, relaxation techniques, and distraction methods that in turn can help alleviate pain and improve sleep. Counselors trained in cognitive behavioral therapy can help in the treatment of insomnia as well.

Antidepressants can help lessen depression and, in some cases, improve sleep and pain. For example, someone with depression who has trouble sleeping may benefit from a selective norepinephrine reuptake inhibitor or a low-dose tricyclic antidepressant. An individual who has trouble with depression and daytime drowsiness not related to sleep might benefit from a selective serotonin reuptake inhibitor.

In treating the older adult for depression, potential side effects must be seriously considered. It is important to review the potential side effects. For example, tricyclic antidepressants have anticholinergic effects, causing constipation and urinary retention, already problems for many older adults. In addition, the sedative effects put older adults at risk for falls, leading to increased mortality and cost. Tricyclic antidepressants are therefore not a first choice for older adults. The elderly often need to have individualized medication plans due to changes in organ systems and the way medications are metabolized, complicating treatment. Consultation with a behavioral health specialist may be beneficial in development of treatment plans to maximize efficacy without increasing side effects.

Sleep

Sleep is an important factor affected by and contributing to the experience of pain. The first step is to eliminate sleep disorders, such as sleep apnea, which can be detected using a combination of tools noted previously. Referral to a sleep specialist or sleep center can aid in appropriate diagnosis and treatment. Once other sleep disorders are adequately treated, remaining problems need to be identified and an appropriate treatment plan needs to be developed. There are several methods to improve sleep, including cognitive behavioral therapy, sleep hygiene, and medications. In older adults, nonpharmacological treatment options are preferred to enhance sleep due to undue side effects of many of the hypnotic medications.

Cognitive Behavior Therapy (CBT)

Cognitive behavioral therapy (CBT) has demonstrated positive results on both sleep and pain. CBT is not only accepted, but also encouraged, in the treatment of insomnia. Two studies found CBT for primary insomnia to be effective in improving sleep continuity with improvements continuing at six months and two years. In addition, the benefits of CBT were as effective as benzodiazepine receptor agonists and hypnotic medications, an attractive option in avoiding medication risks in older adults. There are specially trained individuals who perform CBT training, but all health care professionals can teach the behavioral modifications to patients suffering from pain and sleep disturbance.

Sleep Hygiene

Behaviors to improve sleep include optimizing sleep hygiene with particular emphasis on sleep restriction and stimulus control. Sleep hygiene measures are critical to improving sleep and are outlined in Table 5.1. Sleep restriction involves limiting the time spent in bed to closely reflect time slept. For example, someone who goes to bed at 11:30 P.M., falls asleep at 1:00 A.M., wakes at 3:00 A.M. and is awake for one hour then falls back to sleep and wakes for the day at 8 A.M. is actually sleeping only 6 hours per night but is spending 8½ hours in bed. The goal would be to restrict time in bed to 6–6½ hours per night. The rationale is two-fold. First, it limits time in bed to time sleeping, improving the association between bed and sleep. Second, it helps to consolidate sleep by producing a mild sleep restriction. Once the individual sleeps through the night, the total sleep time is eventually increased to remove the deprivation yet maintain sleep. If sleep becomes disrupted again, then the person needs to return to the last time the individual slept through the night with minimal disruption. For example, the person who sleeps a total of eight hours per night but is awake for 30 minutes during the night may benefit from returning to a total of only 7½ hours to eliminate the 30 minutes awake.

There are several keys to making sleep restriction successful. The patient needs to be willing and able to follow the restriction. Many people will reject sleep restriction if not properly educated, and it needs to be clearly pointed out that the restriction is based on current sleep times, not on the time spent in bed. The timing of sleep needs to be acceptable to the individual. This is typically set by the person's desired wake time. For example, if 8 A.M. is the desired wake time, then bedtime would be 1:30 to 2 A.M. Reviewing current patterns and providing education are vital to success. The individual then needs to establish consistent bedtime routines that are clearly different from day-time routines and occur at least 30 minutes before anticipated bedtime. Some suggestions would include washing up, changing into bedclothes, changing rooms, using dimmer lighting, reading nonstimulating materials, or listening to quiet relaxing music. Bedtime routines are based on personal preference and need to be clearly differentiated from the daytime routine.

Another key success factor in sleep hygiene is ensuring that the person goes to bed only when he or she feels sleepy. Some people will continue their bedtime ritual in bed for 10–15 minutes to help promote sleepiness and the onset of sleep. If the individual is not asleep within 20 minutes, then he or she needs to get out of bed, go to the room where the bedtime routine was started, and repeat that drowsiness-inducing behavior (e.g., reading). If the individual falls asleep but awakens in a couple of hours and is unable to fall back to sleep within 15–20 minutes, he or she needs to get up again and repeat the bedtime routine.

Sleep restriction requires the individual to maintain a consistent wake time, regardless of how much sleep was attained during the night, and avoid day-time napping greater than 20 minutes, eight hours after waking. Once awake, exercise and bright sunlight for approximately 30 minutes will help to further cement changes in circadian patterns that will help induce sleep that evening. This is a difficult concept, because many people believe that if they do not get adequate sleep at night, they should sleep later in the morning to make up for the sleep deficit. In reality, this will perpetuate the problem, because it elimi-nates the consistency and will further lose important zeitgebers that keep the circadian cycle functioning properly.

Another behavioral change in promoting sleep hygiene is stimulus control. Stimulus control is eliminating behaviors that link bed with nonsleep-inducing behaviors. For example, people who have pain will often lie down in the afternoon to rest in an attempt to reduce pain. If the person lies in bed, the mind and body will connect lying in bed with pain. To break this pattern, the person needs to find somewhere other than bed to lie down and relieve pain.

Sleep restriction helps reeducate the body to sleep in bed, establishing a positive routine. The bedroom should be comfortable, including mattress firmness, enough sheets and blankets for temperature control, a comfortable room temperature, adequate darkness, and environmental noise control. Mattress firmness was assessed in a study done by Marin, Cyhan, and Miklos (2006). Their findings indicate that the orthopedic mattress that is firmest actually increased pain while a semi-firm mattress correlated with the lowest pain intensity levels. There was not adequate information regarding aids to help improve mattress comfort (e.g., foam or feather mattress toppers). Cooler temperatures assist in the development of drowsiness and can help maintain sleep as it is more closely related to circadian rhythms. The amount of darkness should allow for enough light to get to the bathroom without injury during the night, but not so bright as to interfere with sleep.

Environmental noise can contribute to waking. Each person has a different noise threshold as well as waking threshold. People who are particularly sound sensitive may require more than one measure to help mask routine noises. Some suggestions include using ear plugs, using white noise from a fan or a white noise machine that plays sounds like rain falling or waves hitting a beach, or using softly playing music. In addition, the bedroom should be used only for sleep and not used as a part of the bedtime routine. Work, watching TV, computer games, and other stimulating activities should be done in other areas to strengthen the relationship between sleep and the bed/bedroom. By controlling bedroom stimulus, the body will eventually associate the bedroom with sleep.

Other sleep hygiene measures that contribute to successful sleep include learning and using various relaxation techniques, setting aside "worry time," and avoiding substances that interfere with sleep such as nicotine, alcohol, caffeine, and other recreational drugs. Relaxation techniques may help in reducing pain and can help induce drowsiness. Techniques vary in complexity, varying from deep breathing to progressive relaxation, and need to be taught and practiced regularly. Many people are so busy during the daytime that the only time left in the day to think about problems and stressors is at night when going to bed. Setting aside time prior to bed allows time to think about those things and "let it go" before sleep. For some people, journaling is an effective measure in reducing stress and worry. Alcohol within a couple of hours of bedtime can result in initially suppressed REM sleep with a rebound of REM sleep noted later in the sleep cycle. Caffeine, nicotine, and stimulants prolong sleep latency and can cause more sleep disruption. Tetrahydrocannabinol (THC), one of the active substances in marijuana, causes suppression of REM sleep and SWS.

There are several considerations to take into account when instituting behavioral changes in the elderly. First is to evaluate his or her current living situation and functional abilities. Recent retirement, death of a spouse, living in a house versus apartment building or other group setting, social activities and hobbies, and functional ability are a few areas that need to be assessed. For example, a recently retired person living in a house, who is recently widowed, will have different issues than someone widowed and retired for several years living in a retirement community. These factors can influence what treatments are instituted and what modifications are used. Second, it is critical to assess beliefs regarding sleep and sleep history. Someone who has been awake during the night for several years may not be bothered by this or may be more resistant to treatment. Finally, an adequate support system can improve compliance with treatment and with evaluation of treatment.

Medications and Sleep Aids

Medications are often used in the treatment of insomnia and sleep disturbance that may be helpful if behavior modifications are inadequate. Hypnotics are used most frequently and are the only medications on the market with the indication for use in sleep. There are two categories of hypnotics, benzodiazepines and nonbenzodiazepines. Benzodiazepines currently available in the United States for use as sleep aids include flurazepam, quazepam, triazolam, estazolam, and temazepam. Nonbenzodiazepines include zolpidem, zaleplon, and eszopiclone. Each drug varies in pharmacokinetics and has its own advantages and disadvantages. The newer nonbenzodiazepines potentially are less addictive and tend to have fewer side effects than the traditional benzodiazepines. Benzodiazepines tend to have a longer half-life and longer effectiveness, but they also have risks such as dizziness, over-sedation, hallucinations, and gait disturbances that may lead to falls and increase mortality in older adults. Benzodiazepines also have the potential to interact with other commonly prescribed medications and are not recommended for use in the elderly. Nonbenzodiazepines should be used with caution and closely monitored.

Pain Treatments to Promote Sleep

Specific modalities for treating pain as it relates to promoting sleep will be discussed here. Please refer to Chapters 7 and 8 for in-depth discussion of these therapies. Adequate treatment of pain can improve both sleep and depression. There are several effective interventions for treatment of pain that will also facilitate sleep. These modalities include cognitive behavior therapy (CBT), biofeedback, massage, heat or cold therapy, and medications. CBT includes coping skills training, self-management strategies for pain reduction, increasing physical activity, and reducing stress. Skills commonly taught include relaxation exercises, distraction, stress management techniques, pacing of activities, and learning more adaptive responses to pain. Handouts help reinforce education and may reduce the number of office visits as well as improve adherence to treatment.

Biofeedback teaches individuals to recognize the body's response to pain and helps to focus on treating those particular areas. For example, someone with headaches located at the back of the head can learn through biofeedback to detect tension in the neck and shoulders. Through biofeedback, an individual can learn techniques to help relax muscles in the shoulders, neck, and head. The more adept the person becomes at detecting this tightness, the earlier he or she can use biofeedback techniques to reduce the pain and induce sleep.

Massage is reported in several studies to be at least partially beneficial in reducing pain and facilitating sleep. There are professionals trained in massage, but persons with pain and their family members can learn basic skills that can be used at home. Massage can be used with heat to improve blood flow. Heat and ice can be helpful adjuncts to other treatments and are often under-recognized for treatment plans. Each individual responds differently to each, and different conditions respond better to each. Extended exposure to heat or cold can cause tissue damage, particularly in older individuals with reduced sensation. The reader is referred to Chapter 7 for in-depth discussion of these modalities and cautions for use in older adults.

Treatment measures outlined above are generally safe and easy to implement. This may be particularly attractive in a population not interested in medication management and in the elderly, for whom multiple medications can increase the risk of adverse reactions or medication interactions.

CONCLUSION

Current research has identified the relationship between pain and sleep. Few studies have examined these issues in the elderly. Depression has also been identified as a factor in both sleep and pain and may significantly influence treatment if not appropriately addressed. Several methods of treatment are available for both pain and sleep. Many treatments are effective for both sleep and pain and can improve quality of life. It is important to consider the impact of depression on pain and sleep, and to ensure that depression is adequately treated. Furthermore, treatments that may be safe in the adult population may need caution in older adults to prevent complications and adverse events.

Additional research is needed to further elucidate the relationships between pain, sleep, and depression and how they are expressed and treated in the older population. Cognitive behavioral therapy has shown promise in the treatment of both sleep and pain management in the elderly population, but further studies are needed to confirm the current results and to identify additional treatment options.

REFERENCES

Aigner, M., Graf, A., Freidl, M., Prause, W., Weiss, M., Kaup-Eder, B., et al. (2003). Sleep disturbance in somatoform pain disorder. *Psychopathology, 36,* 324–328.

Bedard, M. A., Montplaisir, J., Richer, F., Roulou, I., & Malo, J. (1991). Obstructive sleep apnea syndrome: Pathogenesis of neuropsychological deficits. *Journal of Clinical and Experimental Neuropsychology, 13,* 590–964.

Bliwise, D. L. (2000). Normal aging. In M. H. Kryger, T. Roth, & W. C. Dement (Eds.), *Sleep medicine* (pp. 26–42). Philadelphia: W. B. Saunders Company.

Boeve, S. A., Aaron, L. A., Martin-Herz, S. P., Peterson, A., Cain, V., Heimbach, D. M., et al. (2002). Sleep disturbance after burn injury. *Journal of Burn Care and Rehabilitation, 23*(1), 32–38.

Borbely, A. A., & Wirz-Justice, A. (1982). Sleep, sleep deprivation, and depression: A hypothesis derived from a model of sleep regulation. *Human Neurobiology, 1,* 205–210.

Budh, C. N., Hulting, C., & Lundeberg, T. (2005). Quality of sleep in individuals with spinal cord injury: A comparison between patients with and without pain. *Spinal Cord, 43,* 85–95.

Buysse, D. J., Browman, K. E., Monk, T. H., Reynolds, C. F. I. III, Fasiczka, B. A., & Kupfer, D. J. (1992). Napping and 24-hour sleep/wake patterns in healthy elderly and young adults. *Journal of American Geriatrics Society, 40,* 779–786.

Cagnacci, A., Elliott, J. A., & Yen, S.S.C. (1992). Melatonin: A major regulator of the circadian rhythm of core temperature in humans. *Journal of Clinical Endocrinology and Metabolism, 75,* 447–452.

Call-Schmidt, T. A., & Richardson, S. J. (2003). Prevalence of sleep disturbance and its relationship to pain in adults with chronic pain. *Pain Management Nursing, 4*(3), 124–133.

Campbell, S. S., & Zulley, J. (1989). Evidence for circadian influence on human slow wave sleep during daytime sleep episodes. *Psychophysiology, 26,* 580–585.

Carskadon, M. A., & Dement, W. C. (2000). Normal human sleep: An overview. In M. H. Kryger, T. Roth, & W. C. Dement (Eds.), *Sleep medicine* (pp. 15–42). Philadelphia: W. B. Saunders Company.

Cooperman, N. R., Mullin, F. J., & Kleitman, N. (1934). Studies on the physiology of sleep: XI. Further observations on effects of prolonged sleeplessness. *American Journal of Physiology, 107,* 589–593.

Cronin, A. J., Keifer, J. C., Davies, M. F., King, T. S., & Bixler, E. O. (2001). Postoperative sleep disturbance: Influences of opioids and pain in humans. *Sleep, 24*(1), 39–44.

Dinges, D. J., Pack, F., Williams, K., Gillen, K. A., Powell, J. W., Ott, G. E., et al. (1997). Cumulative sleepiness, mood disturbance, and psychomotor vigilance performance decrements during a week of sleep restricted to 4–5 hours per night. *Sleep, 20,* 267–277.

Drewes, A. M., Nielsen, K. D., Arendt-Nielsen, L., Birket-Smith, L., & Hansen, L. M. (1997). The effect of cutaneous and deep pain on the electroencephalogram during sleep: An experimental study. *Sleep, 20*(8), 632–640.

Drewes, A. M., Nielson, K. D., Hansen, B., Taagholt, S. J., Bjerregard, K., & Svendsen, L. (2000). A longitudinal study of clinical symptoms and sleep parameters in rheumatoid arthritis. *Rheumatology, 39,* 1287–1289.

Fielden, J. M., Gander, P. H., Horne, J. G., Lewer, B.M.F., Green, R. M., & Devane, P. A. (2003). An assessment of sleep disturbance in patients before and after total hip arthroplasty. *Journal of Arthroplasty, 18*(3), 371–376.

Foley, D. J., Monjan, A. A., Brown, S. L., Simonsick, E. M., Wallace, R. B., & Blazer, D. G. (1995). Sleep complaints among elderly persons: An epidemiologic study of three communities. *Sleep, 18,* 425–432.

Friedman, J., Globus, G., & Huntley, A. (1977). Performance and mood during and after gradual sleep reduction. *Psychophysiology, 14,* 245–250.

Ganguli, M., Reynolds, C. F., & Gilby, J. E. (1996). Prevalence and persistence of sleep complaints in rural older community sample: The MoVIES project. *Journal of American Geriatrics Society, 44,* 778–784.

Hirshkowitz, M., Moore, C. A., Hamilton, C.R.I., Rando, K. C., & Karacan, I. (1992). Polysomnography of adults and elderly: sleep architecture, respirations, and leg movement. *Journal of Clinical Neurophysiology, 9*(1), 56–62.

Koopman, C., Nouriani, B., Erickson, B. A., Anupindi, R., Butler, L. D., Bachmann, M. H., et al. (2002). Sleep disturbance in women with metastatic breast cancer. *The Breast Journal, 8*(6), 362–370.

Landis, C. A., Levine, J. D., & Robinson, C. R. (1988). Decreased slow-wave and paradoxical sleep in a rat chronic pain model. *Sleep, 12*(2), 167–177.

Lentz, M. J., Landis, C. A., Rothermel, J., & Shaver, J. I. (1999). Effects of selective slow wave sleep disruption on musculoskeletal pain and fatigue in middle aged women. *Journal of Rheumatology, 26,* 1586–1592.

Lobbezoo, F., Visscher, C. M., & Naeije, M. (2003). Impaired health status, sleep disorders, and pain in the craniomandibular and cervical spinal regions. *European Journal of Pain, 8,* 23–30.

Marin, R., Cyhan, T., & Miklos, W. (2006). Sleep disturbance in patients with chronic low back pain. *American Journal of Physical Medicine and Rehabilitation, 85*(5), 430–435.

Moldofsky, H., & Scarisbrick, P. (1976). Induction of neurasthenic musculoskeletal pain syndrome by selective sleep stage deprivation. *Psychosomatic Medicine, 38*(1), 35–44.

Monk, T. H., Buysse, D. J., Carrier, J., Billy, B. D., & Rose, L. R. (2001). Effects of afternoon siesta naps on sleep, alertness, performance, and circadian rhythms in the elderly. *Sleep, 24,* 680–687.

Myers, B. L., & Badia, P. (1995). Changes in circadian rhythms and sleep quality with aging: Mechanisms and interventions. *Neurosciences and Biobehavioral Reviews, 19,* 553–571.

Naylor, E., Penev, P. D., Orbeta, L., Janssen, I., Ortiz, R., Colecchia, E. F., et al. (2000). Daily social and physical activity increases slow wave sleep and daytime neuropsychological performance in the elderly. *Sleep, 23*(1), 87–95.

Onen, S. H., Alloui, A., Gross, A., Eschallier, A., & Dubray, C. (2001). The effects of total sleep deprivation, selective sleep interruption and sleep recovery on pain tolerance thresholds in healthy subjects. *Journal of Sleep Research, 10,* 35–42.

Pilcher, J. J., & Huffcutt, A. I. (1996). Effects of sleep deprivation on performance: A meta-analysis study. *Sleep, 13,* 410–424.

Pilowsky, I., Crettenden, I., & Townley, M. (1985). Sleep disturbance in pain clinic patients. *Pain, 23,* 27–33.

Smith, M. T., & Haythornthwaite, J. A. (2003). How do sleep disturbance and chronic pain inter-relate? Insights from the longitudinal and cognitive-behavioral clinical traits literature. *Sleep Medicine Reviews, 8,* 119–132.

Wilcox, S., Brenes, G. A., Levine, D., Sevick, M. A., Shumaker, S. A., & Craven, T. (2000). Factors related to sleep disturbance in older adults experiencing knee pain or knee pain with radiographic evidence of knee osteoarthritis. *Journal of the American Geriatrics Society, 48*(10), 1241–1251.

Wittig, R. M., Zorick, F. J., Blumer, D., Heilbronn, M., & Roth, T. (1982). Disturbed sleep in patients complaining of chronic pain. *Journal of Nervous and Mental Disorders, 170,* 429–431.

SECTION II

Multidisciplinary Approach to Pain Management in the Older Adult

CHAPTER 6

Multimodality Approach to Pain Management

Michaelene P. Jansen

The first section of this book focuses on understanding and assessing pain in older adults. The purpose of the second section of the book is to provide the reader with a broad perspective of available treatment options. This chapter presents an overview of the treatment options and rationale for a multimodality/multidisciplinary approach to pain. The treatment of pain is very challenging for the patient, provider, and family. How to best optimize function and mobility while reducing the pain and limiting adverse effects of the treatment is not an easy task. The treatment of pain in the older adult adds another layer of complexity to this monumental task. The older adult may suffer not only from pain, but also several chronic illnesses, family stresses, and financial hardship, all of which contribute to pain perception. Providing more than one treatment option is vital to the success of any pain management approach.

Treating any chronic illness or disease presents a challenge for health care professionals, in that a single treatment or agent will rarely control symptoms. Most chronic conditions require multiple strategies to prevent progression or to control the disease (Clark, McAlister, Hartling, & Vandermeer, 2005). For example, a patient with hypertension will need standard treatment, which includes lifestyle modifications such as weight loss, diet changes, and smoking cessation along with one or more pharmacologic agents. A single pharmacologic agent without lifestyle modifications is rarely successful in managing hypertension. The treatment for pain in an older adult is no exception.

A multimodality approach to pain may consist of many dimensions. A multimodal approach to pain incorporates genetic, molecular, physiological, emotional, and sociocultural factors. The authors would like to challenge the reader to think more broadly in utilizing multiple treatment options. In addition to the numerous modalities available to the provider, other aspects of care need to be considered in formulating a comprehensive plan. For example, understanding how gender differences affect the brain and behavior may be as important as finding the right nonpharmacologic and pharmacologic strategies. For example, there has been some evidence that gender differences have an effect in the pharmacological effects of medications (Becker, Arnold, Berkley, Blaustein, Eckel, et al., 2005). Cultural issues have also shown to play a role in pain severity and treatment (Reyes-Gibby, Aday, Todd, Cleeland, & Anderson, 2007).

DEVELOPING A COMPREHENSIVE PAIN MANAGEMENT PLAN

All providers are able to develop a comprehensive pain management plan for older adults, but often do not feel comfortable in doing so. Many patients are referred to pain centers that provide a comprehensive approach to pain. Ideally, the pain centers work closely with primary care providers to insure a comprehensive treatment plan that is manageable for the patient. A common theme throughout the literature on multimodal approaches to chronic illnesses is to individualize the plan for the patient to improve compliance and efficacy of treatment. Primary care providers provide the crucial link in helping patients individualize their treatment plan in adhering to the pain management plan. An overall goal of treatment is to achieve or maintain quality of life. Function, pleasure, and independence are integral in reaching that goal for the older adult.

The use of both nonpharmacologic and pharmacologic treatments have shown to result in greater reductions in pain and increased functional ability (Ferrell & Ferrell, 1996; Podichetty, Mazanec, & Biscup, 2003). Table 6.1 provides a list of treatment options that have demonstrated effectiveness in reducing pain. There is evidence of endogenous opioid release, which is associated with pain modulation with several of the interventions discussed in the next several chapters.

Function

One of the frustrating aspects of managing pain is to determine how to fully assess the effectiveness of any intervention. In treating acute pain, primarily

TABLE 6.1   Therapy Options for Pain Management

Somatic Interventions	Situational	Medications
Heat/cold	Education	NSAIDs
Exercise	Attitude	Acetaminophen
Massage	Meditation	Opioids
Relaxation	Aromatherapy	Antidepressants
Physical therapy	Hypnosis	Anticonvulsants
Traction	Biofeedback	GABA agonists
Manipulation	Support/advocacy groups	Serotonin agonists
TENS	Individual and family counseling	Alpha 2 agonists
Acupuncture	Cognitive therapy	
Local anesthetics	Behavioral therapy	
Dorsal column stimulation	Hobbies	
Nerve blocks	Networking	
Local ganglion blocks		
Sympathectomy		
Rhizotomy		
Deep brain stimulation		

with pharmacologic interventions, pain is assessed by utilizing a numerical rating scale before and after intervention. However, as Chapter 3 points out, with persistent pain, the numerical rating scale may not be the most appropriate assessment for older adults. For example, a patient may rate their hip pain as a 7 (on a 0–10 scale) prior to institution of physical therapy, analgesic medications, and healing touch. At a follow-up appointment, they may still rate their pain as a 7 (on a 0–10 scale); yet with a functional assessment, it is found that the older person's sleep is uninterrupted, and; they are able to participate in social activities and use assistive devices less frequently. Without utilizing a functional component of assessment, the provider may assume that the pain is not managed adequately and inappropriately increase the analgesic medication for that older adult.

The American Chronic Pain Association has developed the Quality of Life Scale to help individuals measure their activity levels over time (Cowan & Kelly, 2003). The scale ranges from 0–10 like the numeric pain scale but has a level of activity associated with each number. The score of the scale, however, is the inverse of the pain scale. For example, a 0 indicates that the person lies in bed all day and feels hopeless and helpless. A score of 10 indicates that the person has normal outside activity and active social and family life.

Nonpharmacologic Treatments

Nonpharmacologic interventions should be an integral part of any pain management plan (Middaugh & Pawlick, 2002; Podichetty, Mazanec, & Biscup, 2003). Chapters 7 and 8 outline numerous therapies and interventions that have shown effectiveness in treating pain. Several therapies can be performed by the individual. Other therapies need to be performed by licensed and certified therapists. The following chapters provide an excellent overview of the various therapies, with recommendations specific to older adults.

Physical therapy, in particular, provides numerous options for pain management. Some patients may initially decline a physical therapy referral because they have tried it before and found it was not effective. However, the patient needs to be aware that various methods can improve function and mobility and that a new series of therapy may be beneficial. Older adults in particular can benefit from physical therapy in many ways. Muscle strengthening, balance, and gait are useful in preventing falls due to arthritis or limited mobility. Many older adults suffer from greater trochanter bursitis that can occur from adjusting their gait secondary to degenerative spine disease. Iontopheresis can reduce the inflammation and pain associated with this condition.

Exercise continues to be a consistent variable in the improvement of pain over time. Chapter 7 provides evidence and support for ongoing exercise programs in achieving the goal of reduced pain and reversing physical impairments. Exercise improves range of motion, thus increasing strength and power, providing postural and gait stability. All exercise should improve flexibility, strength, and endurance. Exercise programs supporting these concepts have become more available in communities and through media in recent years.

Warm water exercises or aqua therapy may also benefit older adults. This therapy is described in further detail in Chapter 7 but deserves some extra attention here. The buoyancy of the water puts less pressure on joints and facilitates movement. The disadvantage of aqua therapy for older adults is that many communities do not have public pools or programs available locally. Many insurance programs only cover therapy programs run by a certified therapist for a set amount of time.

Chiropractic care is not specifically discussed in this text, but its benefits need to be acknowledged. Many patients with mechanical back pain can obtain relief from chiropractic treatments. One study in particular examined six weeks of chiropractic treatment and dietary supplements for persistent pain, primarily low back pain, in adults over age 55 (Hawk, Long, Boulanger, Morschlauser, & Fuhr, 2000). Their findings showed improvement in the Pain Disability Index and decreased use of pain medications. Although this study supports the use of chiropractic treatment, the authors recommend further study in older adults.

The use of complementary and alternative therapies is increasing among all age levels. Traditional medicine does not always provide the desired outcome for patients. Alternative or less invasive therapies provide an additional option for patients. The creation of the National Center for Complementary and Alternative Medicine (NCCAM) within the National Institutes of Health has provided an avenue and funding for scientific research on complementary and alternative therapies. The center also provides useful information and reviews on complementary and alternative therapies. For example, the center recently compiled a review based on scientific evidence on the effectiveness of complementary and alternative therapies in the treatment of rheumatoid arthritis (National Center for Complementary and Alternative Medicine, 2006).

Cognitive and behavior strategies are also important in the overall pain management plan. There is some evidence supporting the idea that personality in young adulthood can predict persistent pain conditions in midlife and older adulthood (Applegate, Keefe, Siegler, Bradley, McKee, et al., 2005). Cognitive and behavioral therapy can modify helplessness and low self-esteem. Negative coping, such as the perception of pain as catastrophic, and events associated with pain can also be reduced with cognitive and behavior therapy (AGS, 2002).

Education of providers and patients cannot be overemphasized. Providers can become more proficient in the recognition, evaluation, and management of pain if they have received adequate pain education in their training and continuing education programs (Chen, Goodman, Galicia-Castillo, Quidgley-Nevares, Krebs, et al., 2007; Winn & Dentino, 2004). Patient education and self-management skills have also demonstrated support for improving function and pain in older adults (Ersek, Turner, McCurry, Gibbons, & Kraybill, 2003).

Pharmacologic Therapies

Pharmacologic therapy for pain in older adults is the most common therapy used. The literature supports utilizing nonpharmacologic therapies in conjunction with analgesic medications. The use of multiple therapies in managing pain has shown a decrease in drug doses over time (AGS, 2002). A combination of two or more drugs may have complementary or synergistic effect with less risk of adverse reactions or toxicity than a higher dose of a single drug (AGS, 2002). However, in older adults, pharmacologic intervention needs to be evaluated very carefully due to physiological effects of age on the liver and kidneys. Chapter 9 provides an in-depth discussion of medications used in the treatment of pain in older adults. The risk versus benefits of the various types of medications is evaluated under each category of medication. Special attention is paid to polypharmacology in the older adult. Reducing drug interactions, along with limiting adverse events, is a goal in developing a pain management plan for an older adult.

Persistent pain is often undertreated in older adults, because providers either believe that painful conditions are a part of aging, or because there is concern with the safety of administering analgesics in older adults, particularly those over 85 years old. Chapter 9 examines this issue very carefully and provides evidence that analgesic medications can be safely prescribed for older adults. Lower doses of medications can be prescribed when used in conjunction of other nonpharmacologic therapies.

Interventional Therapies

Interventional therapies have shown benefit in managing pain in older adults, particularly pain related to degenerative disease that has a radicular component. Chapter 10 describes a variety of interventions that can be used. Most, if not all of these interventions should be performed by a pain specialist under fluoroscopic visualization.

Long term interventions discussed in Chapter 10 include implantable spinal cord stimulators and implantable intrathecal pumps. Expanded indications for use and development of new types of spinal cord stimulators hold promise for this mode of therapy. Long-term use of intrathecal pumps has received mixed reviews over the years, yet this modality shows merit in many persistent pain or spastic conditions. The use of intrathecal baclofen is gaining more acceptance in a variety of neurological arenas.

SUMMARY

This chapter provides a brief overview of the various types of pain management strategies for older adults. The focus of this chapter is to emphasize the importance of utilizing multiple strategies and therapies in formulating a comprehensive pain management plan for older adults. The use of multiple therapies for controlling pain has shown to reduce the number or dose of medications used. This is an important concept in managing pain in older adults. The goal of therapy is to increase function, reduce pain, and improve quality of life, because persistent pain is rarely completely eliminated.

REFERENCES

American Geriatric Society (AGS). (2002). The management of persistent pain in older persons. AGS Panel on Persistent Pain in Older Persons. *Journal of the American Geriatric Society, 50*(6 Suppl.), S205–S224.

Applegate, K. L., Keefe, F. J., Siegler, I. C., Bradley, L. A., McKee, D. C., Cooper, K. S., et al. (2005). Does personality at college entry predict number of reported pain conditions at mid-life? A longitudinal study. *The Journal of Pain, 6,* 92–97.

Becker, J. B., Arnold, A. P., Berley, K. J., Blaustein, J. D., Eckel, L. A., Hampson, E., et al. (2005). Strategies and methods for research on sex differences in brain and behavior. *Endocrinology, 146,* 1650–1673.

Chen, I., Goodman, B., Galicia-Castillo, M., Quidgley-Nevares, A., Krebs, M., & Gliva-McConvey, G. (2007). The EVMS pain education initiative: A multifaceted approach to resident education. *The Journal of Pain, 8,* 152–160.

Clark, A. M., McAlister, F. A., Hartling, L., & Vandermeer, B. (2005). Randomized trials of secondary prevention programs in coronary artery disease: A systematic review. Agency for Health Care Research and Quality. *American Geriatric Society, 50,* S205–S224.

Cowan, P., & Kelly, N. (2003). American Chronic Pain Association Quality of Life Scale. Retrieved December 30, 2007, from www.theacpa.org/documents/Quality_of_Life_Scale.pdf.

Ersek, M., Turner, J. A., McCurry, S. M., Gibbons, L., & Kraybill, B. M. (2003). Efficacy of a self-management group intervention for elderly persons with chronic pain. *The Clinical Journal of Pain, 19,* 156–167.

Ferrell, B. R., & Ferrell, B. A., Eds. (1996). *Pain in the elderly.* Seattle: IASP Press.

Hawk, C., Long, C. R., Boulanger, K. T., Morschlauser, E., & Fuhr, A. W. (2000). Chiropractic care for patients aged 55 years and older: Report from practice-based research. *Journal of the American Geriatrics Society, 48,* 534–545.

Middaugh, S. J., & Pawlick, K. (2002). Biofeedback and behavioral treatment of persistent pain in the older adult: A review and a study. *Applied Psychophysiology and Biofeedback, 27,* 185–202.

National Center for Complementary and Alternative Medicine. (2006). Rheumatoid arthritis and complementary and alternative medicine. Retrieved December 30, 2007, from http://nccam.nih.gov/health/RA/.

Podichetty, V. K., Mazanec, D. J., & Biscup, R. S. (2003). Chronic non-malignant musculoskeletal pain in older adults: clinical issues and opioid intervention. *Postgraduate Medical Journal, 79*(937), 627–633.

Reyes-Gibby, C. C., Aday, L. A., Todd, K. H., Cleeland, C. S., & Anderson, K. O. (2007). Pain in aging community-dwelling adults in the United States: Non-Hispanic whites, non-Hispanic blacks and Hispanics. *The Journal of Pain, 8*(1), 75–84.

Winn, P. A., & Dentino, A. N. (2004). Effective pain management in the long-term care setting. *Journal of the American Medical Directors Association, 5*(5), 342–352.

CHAPTER 7

Physical Therapy

Michele Komp-Webb

Persistent pain in older adults often involves the musculoskeletal system, resulting in loss of mobility, restriction in joint motion, or altered balance and gait. Persistent pain will result in decreased activity in a population that is already predominately inactive and will increase the possibility of social isolation and depression (Gibson, Katz, Corran, Farrell, & Helme, 1994). The painful body part will become weaker and total body deconditioning will occur (Roesch & Ulrich, 1980).

There is a strong belief among some experts that physiological changes that occur with aging can result in a decreased ability to perceive pain. Thermal stimulation must be 20%–80% greater before it is felt in the geriatric subject versus a younger subject (Gibson et al., 1994; Harkins, Price, & Martelli, 1986). The intensity of stimulation required to trigger a withdrawal response is higher (Harkins et al., 1986; Gibson et al., 1994). One study revealed slower cognitive functioning as a result of changes to the central nervous system. Middaugh and colleagues (1998) reported that geriatric patients could benefit from chronic pain programs as much as if not more than younger patients. Physical modalities and exercise should be at the core of any approach toward managing pain in the geriatric population (Gloth & Matesi, 2001a). Physical relief of musculoskeletal pain, chronic or acute, will not last long unless accompanied by exercise that will alter the source of pain.

Physical therapists assist patients in understanding the difference between "hurt" and "harm." Activities may cause discomfort or hurt but that does not mean damage or harm is being done to the body. Persons with chronic pain have sensitized nervous systems, meaning that even normal stimuli, such as gentle touch, can trigger a painful response. During the acute pain stage, immediately after injury, the body warns us to not do further damage by triggering a pain response. Over time, this response becomes overtaxed and simply tells the now chronic pain sufferer the wrong information. Diagnostic images can tell us what is wrong, but not what hurts. A large disc bulge in one patient can cause no pain in one individual and excruciating pain for another. The evaluation of symptoms and response to hands-on testing will tell the physical therapist more than most diagnostic studies. However, by no means is the information from diagnostic testing disregarded. The information provided by various diagnostic studies is combined with all other aspects of the patient's care to formulate an appropriate treatment plan.

Physical therapist and physical therapist assistants have many tools to assist the older population with pain relief and improving functional mobility, balance, strength, endurance, and independence. Studies of the treatment modalities reviewed in this chapter reveal limited but positive evidence of their effectiveness in treating chronic pain in older adults. Specific physical agents (e.g., ultrasound, ice) are not to be used as the only approach for the treatment of pain. The American Physical Therapy Association wrote in 1995, "Without documentation which justifies the necessity of the exclusive use of physical agents/modalities, the use of physical agents/modalities, in the absence of other skilled therapeutic or educational intervention, should not be considered physical therapy" (Allen, 2006). Interestingly, the modality with the greatest support for pain management is therapeutic exercise (Rakel & Barr, 2003).

The following discussion describes common physical therapy procedures and treatments. Although there have been recent developments in physical therapy treatment, many of the therapies have been used for decades. Many of the references will reflect the longevity and historical nature of these therapies.

TREATMENT MODALITIES

Superficial Heating

Superficial heating is used for pain relief, deceasing muscle spasms (Baker & Bell, 1991), increasing blood flow locally due to vasodilatation, increasing relaxation, and preparing stiff muscles and joints for exercise (Baker & Bell, 1991; Borrell et al., 1980). Heat can act as a counter-irritant as it will change the sensory input to the skin, blocking pain perception and the tissue's response to it. Heat will decrease the sensitivity of trigger points. Superficial heat will penetrate 1–2 cm deep, affecting the skin and superficial subcutaneous tissues (Michlovitz, 1990). Examples of superficial heat include hydrocollator packs, paraffin baths, fluidotherapy, hydrotherapy, and short-wave diathermy. Each of these modalities will be discussed in further detail.

Indications

Superficial heat is used to decrease generalized pain and pain associated with bursitis, tendonitis, trigger points, muscle spasm, fibromyalgia, myofascial pain, headaches, and osteoarthritis. There is some belief that during nonactive stages of rheumatoid arthritis, patients will experience relief with superficial heat. Those who have back and cervical pain respond well, but temporarily, to heating.

Physiologic Effects

Increasing the temperature of collagen will enhance its elastic properties and improve its response to stretch (Collins, Storey, & Peterson, 1986). Heat will increase collagenase activity, improving healing (Perret, Rim, & Cristan, 2006), and overall decrease joint stiffness. Local blood flow will increase and carry more oxygen to tissues, increasing metabolism (Lee, Itoh, Yany, & Eason, 1990; Gloth & Matesi, 2001b). This in turn promotes healing, restores proper nutrition, and eliminates waste products (Lee, Itoh, Yany, & Eason, 1990). Heat will decrease chronic inflammation but will increase acute inflammation and edema and increase bleeding. Heat can decrease pain by elevating the pain threshold (Lehmann, Brunner, & Stow, 1958; Wadsworth & Chanmugam, 1988), altering sensory nerve conduction velocity (Abramson et al., 1996; Lee et al., 1990; Halle et al., 1981; Lee, Rexrode, Cook, Hennekines, & Burin, 2001), and changing the rate of muscle spindle firing (Mense, 1978).

Superficial heat will act as a counterirritant and promote general relaxation. Vasodiliation will occur, and this combined, with increased cell membrane permeability, results in washing out pain mediators in the bloodstream. The gate control theory of pain also contributes to the perception of decreased pain. The gate control theory states that small-diameter, slow-conducting nociceptive nerve fibers transmit painful stimuli to the spinal cord. This stimulation is then sent to the brain. These slow fibers can be inhibited by large-diameter, fast-conducting sensory nerve fibers. Heating will stimulate the sensory nerve fibers, inhibiting the pain signal to the brain.

Precautions and Contraindications

Care should be taken when treating older adults with decreased skin sensitivity, impaired cognition, and heat intolerance. Individuals with bleeding disorders, inherent or medically induced, should be monitored closely. Open areas must be covered, especially when using a paraffin bath. Specific precautions to each modality are mentioned further in this chapter.

Heat should never be used on individuals demonstrating acute inflammation, trauma, or circulatory compromise; over a region of malignancy; those on anticoagulant therapy; and those with severe sensory or cognitive impairments (Lee et al., 1990). Patients with multiple sclerosis generally have a poor tolerance to heating by full body immersion. Contraindications listed specifically for fluidotherapy include hepatitis, chicken pox, typhoid, paratyphoid, sepsis, or other infectious diseases (Herrick & Herrick, 1992). People with open areas that cannot be completely covered should not be treated with paraffin baths. Paraffin baths should not be used with those who have a rash, local infection, or dermatitis (Lee et al., 1990). Other superficial heating agents can be used with less incidence of contamination. Some sources believe that heat should not be used on those with active rheumatoid arthritis.

Reimbursement

Very few insurance companies will pay for hot packs. All other superficial heat modalities are usually covered benefits.

Types of Superficial Heating

Hydrocollator packs/hot packs. Hot packs are usually hydrophylic silicate dioxide sand-filled packs kept in hot water at temperatures between 158–167°F/70–80°C. The sand can absorb many times its weight in water, producing a gel-like substance that is easy to conform to body parts. Six to eight cotton towel layers must be applied between the skin and the hot pack to prevent burning. This wet heat will penetrate deeper than dry heat. Application is for 15–20 minutes and therapeutic temperature is held for 20–30 minutes (Perret et al., 2006). Heat wraps, a new form of heat to manage chronic pain, are purchased over the counter and worn for up to eight hours. Several studies found pain is decreased for a longer period of time following the wearing of heat wraps versus brief heating through hot packs (O'Connor & McCarberg, 2005).

Heating pads. Older adults often use heating pads to decrease pain in joints and muscles. The target heat level is 125°F/52°C, but temperatures fluctuate widely. Given the frail skin, peripheral neuropathy, and impaired cognition that may be present in older adults, extreme caution should be used in recommending this home remedy for older adults. Many adults, both young and old, have fallen asleep with heating pads on their skin, resulting in partial thickness burns.

Paraffin baths. Paraffin baths are a combination of wax and oil kept at 113–129°F/45–54°C. They are best used for the distal extremities. The affected body part is dipped into the melted paraffin several times, wrapped in a plastic bag, and then wrapped with towels. The wax is left on for up to 20 minutes. The wax can be painted onto body areas that cannot be dipped. Besides increasing tissue temperature, the oil will lubricate and condition the skin. This is an excellent modality for treating rheumatoid arthritis and joint contractures of the hands. Home units are available.

Fluidotherapy. Fluidotherapy transfers heat to an extremity using forced convection. Warm air, heated to 115–120°F/46.1–48.9°C, is circulated uniformly through a container filled with cellex, finely ground corncob. The affected extremity is placed into a sleeve connected to the inside of the container. The resultant sensation is that of a solid acting like a fluid, or like a "dry whirlpool." The affected limb is levitated and receives a massaging action that provides sensory stimulation and relaxation (Herrick & Herrick, 1992). The temperature and the amount of agitation of the cellex can be altered for patient comfort and treatment goals. The patient can perform range-of-motion exercises during treatment. Fluidotherapy is appropriate for those with open wounds as long as they are completely covered. One study demonstrated that fluidotherapy was superior to ultrasound, paraffin wax, and whirlpool in increasing tissue temperature .5–1.2 cm below the skin (Borrel et al., 1980).

Hydrotherapy. Hydrotherapy or whirlpool treatments are the oldest method for managing pain and musculoskeletal dysfunction. There are a variety of tank sizes and shapes to accommodate specific body parts; the highboy for submersion of upper extremities or feet, up to the very large, butterfly-shaped Hubbard tank for full body immersion. There are freestanding mini-pools that allow for upright body immersion for exercises, which utilize much less space than a therapy pool. All whirlpool tanks have a turbine engine for water agitation. The direction and intensity of the agitation can be adjusted to assist or resist exercise or to provide wound debridement. Duration of treatment is for 20 minutes in water temperatures of 97.1–104.9°F/36.5–40.5°C. Cleaning the tanks between each patient is of utmost importance to prevent contamination and infection. Most manufacturers supply instruction and chemical additives. Precautions and contraindications are different depending on whether full to near-full body immersion is indicated, and these guidelines are listed previously under contraindications.

Short-wave Diathermy. Short-wave diathermy is a therapy that is not commonly used. The patient is placed within an electromagnetic field created by high-frequency alternating currents (Lee et al., 1990). The patient's tissues will resist the current creating heat. Heat penetration is to 1–2 centimeters. There are many contraindications and precautions specific to this modality that makes it less desirable than others listed.

Cryotherapy

The purpose of cryotherapy is to decrease pain, edema, inflammation, and muscle spasms. Prior to exercise, cryotherapy will temporarily decrease spasticity, defined as an increased response to passive stretch, increased deep-tendon reflexes, and clonus. Examples include cold packs, ice massage, cold baths or whirlpools, vapocoolant sprays, and cold compression units. Each modality will be described in further detail.

Indications

Diagnoses that respond well to cryotherapy include trigger points, acute edema, muscle spasm, acute musculoskeletal injuries (sprains and strains), tendonitis, bursitis, spasticity found in stroke patients and those with cerebral palsy, joint replacements, myofascial pain syndrome, and fibromyalgia. Incidentally, there is no consensus on the effectiveness of cold versus heat for pain control (Lee et al., 1990). Cold therapy is indicated over heat therapy for acute injuries but otherwise decisions should be made based on patient comfort and treatment protocols.

Physiologic effects

After an injury, the body releases vasoactive agents, such as histamine. These agents mediate inflammation by allowing fluid leakage into the interstitium (Fox & Wyatt, 1962; Michlovitz, 1990). Cryotherapy will decrease this response via vasoconstriction and by directly decreasing the vasoactive agents in the treated area. Cryotherapy will decrease pain by elevating the pain threshold via alterations in nerve conduction velocity (Lee et al., 1990; Lee, Warren, & Mason, 1978). There may be a decrease in narcotic use as a result of decreased pain (Conolly, Paltos, & Tooth, 1972). Cooling tissue reduces skeletal muscle spasm by decreasing the activity of muscle spindles and the peripheral nerves (Lee et al., 1990). Muscle fatigue will be decreased (Perret et al., 2006). Spasticity will be decreased via a mechanism that is not well understood but appears to be due to prolonged cooling of muscle spindles (Hartvikksen, 1962; Perret et al., 2006). Studies have indicated that cooling of a normally functioning muscle prior to exercise may enhance performance (Perkins, Li, & Nicholas, 1950). Joint stiffness increases due to increased tissue viscosity and a decrease in collagen elasticity. Care needs to be taken not to apply cold therapies for longer than 15 minutes. If a treated area is very cold or is cooled for too long, vasoconstriction is offset by vasodilatation (Clark et al., 1958; Cobbold & Lewis, 1956; Major, Schwinghamer, & Winston, 1981). This post-cooling level of vasodilatation does not return the tissue to its baseline temperature. Extreme cold may result in increased edema and tissue damage (Collins et al., 1986; Perkins et al., 1950; Matsen, Questd, & Matsen, 1975).

Precautions and Contraindications

Patients with hypertension may have an increase in diastolic and systolic blood pressure and need to be monitored closely if a large body area is being cooled. Cooling open wounds may delay healing. Special attention needs to be given to older adults who have impaired circulation, a thermoregulatory disorder, or hypersensitivity to cold. There has been documentation of prolonged nerve damage when ice was applied for several hours over a superficial nerve (Collins et al., 1986). Those who are cognitively impaired or have impaired sensation should be monitored closely.

Cold should never be used to treat individuals with cold uticaria, cryogubulinemia, Raynaud's syndrome, paroxysmal cold hemoglobinuria, compromised circulation (arterial insufficiency), or an anesthetic area (Lee et al., 1990; Michlovitz, 1990).

Reimbursement

Cold packs are rarely a covered benefit. Coverage for other cryotherapy modalities varies by insurance carrier.

Types of Cold Application

Cold packs. Cold packs are silica-gel–filled packs stored at 23°F/–5°C. They are applied to the affected area for 10 to 15 minutes. A cloth layer is placed between the pack and the patient's skin to avoid injury and promote hygiene. A wet cloth will promote cold conduction better than a dry cloth.

Ice massage. Ice massage is applied with formed ice in constant motion. Smaller to mid-sized treatment regions will require 5–10 minutes of icing or until the patient goes through the four sensory stages of intense cold, burning, aching, and analgesia. Active range of motion exercises can be combined with ice massage to improve function.

Cold baths. Cold baths or whirlpools are most often used to treat edematous distal extremities. The temperature should be maintained at 55–64°F/13–18°C. The patient is encouraged to move the involved extremity continuously to assist in "pumping" excessive fluid from the area. Treatment lasts for 10–15 minutes, and older adults need to be closely monitored due to preexisting decreased peripheral circulation.

Vapocoolant sprays. Vapocoolant sprays, made of fluori-methane, are used to treat trigger points or restricted muscles. The restricted muscle is held in a passive stretch while the spray is applied from the proximal to the distal end along the length of the muscle. Fluori-methane was banned in 1990 by the Clean Air Act but received a medical exemption (Michlovitz, 1990). This technique is often called "spray and stretch."

Cold compression units. Cold compression units are often used postoperatively. Some units use gravity to allow iced water to flow from a cooler into a sleeve that fits snugly over the affected area. Once the water warms, it can be drained from the sleeve back into the cooler, mixed with the ice and returned to the sleeve. Others units have pumps that keep the cool water circulating constantly.

Ultrasound

Ultrasound therapy is considered a form of deep heat. It displays thermal and nonthermal effects discussed later in this section. It is used for pain relief, muscle relaxation, subacute edema reduction, increasing collagen/tissue extensibility, and promoting wound healing.

Indications

Ultrasound is used to treat soft tissue pain such as bursitis, tendonitis, trigger points, and muscle spasm. Specific studies indicate positive results when treating lateral epicondylitis (Trudel et al., 2004), calcific tendonitis, adhesive capsulitis, and rotator cuff tendonitis. It will decrease extensive bruising in the subacute phase of healing. It may be applied to decrease subacute edema, pain from neuromas following amputation (McCarberg & O'Connor, 2004), pain from herpes zoster and post-herpetic neuralgia (Payne, 1984), and symptoms from chronic regional pain syndrome (Gloth & Metesi, 2001b). Ultrasound treatments will affect deep joints, tendon sheaths, fibrous scars, and myofascial tissue (Perret et al., 2006). Individuals with low back pain demonstrate improved functional mobility (Ansari et al., 2006) after treatment with ultrasound.

Physiological Effects

Ultrasound will decrease pain in soft tissue by a process that is not well understood. It will increase motor-nerve conduction and decrease sensory and pain nerve conduction (Currier & Kramer, 1982; Edwards et al., 1978; Robertson, 2002). Moore and colleagues (2000) confirmed alteration in nerve latencies and further deduced that these alterations are due to thermal effects and not the nonthermal or mechanical effects of ultrasound. In theory, the pain threshold will be elevated by a decrease in the sensitivity of large diameter fibers, altering pain transmission and thereby supporting the gate control theory (Falconer, Hayes, & Chang, 1990; Halle et al., 1981).

Ultrasound stimulates the large-diameter sensory fibers to decrease the sensation of pain. Pain is decreased by the inhibition of sympathetic activity, stimulation of free nerve endings, and decreasing sensitivity of trigger points. The heat generated with ultrasound will act as a counter-irritant to pain (Kramer, 1984). Ultrasound will increase cutaneous blood flow both by its mechanism of action and by the massaging motion of the ultrasound head (Nobel, Lee, & Griffin-Nobel, 2007). Pain mediators are flushed from the bloodstream from the increase in blood flow (Falconer et al., 1990).

Ultrasound can be used to promote tissue repair by enhancing cell proliferation and protein synthesis. In the context of wound healing, this topic is beyond the scope of this chapter, but ultrasound can be very beneficial in promoting healing. In context of muscle tissue injury, ultrasound appears to decrease the secondary effects of muscle damage by oxidative injury (Freitas, et al., 2006).

The mechanisms by which ultrasound decreases muscle spasms is not well understood but appear to be related to the thermal effects of ultrasound. Theories include a decrease in muscle fiber firing, a decrease in the firing of the golgi tendon organ and Type II nerve fibers, resulting in muscle relaxation (Mense, 1978). A decrease in pain will reflexively result in muscle relaxation.

Ultrasound will increase tissue extensibility and the range of motion of contracted joints prior to stretching (LeBan, 1962; Lehmann et al., 1958; Wright & Johns, 1961). Dense scar tissue will absorb sound waves and heat more readily than surrounding tissue. This results in collagen fiber separation, which makes the scar tissue easier to mobilize and break down. Ultrasound also alters the cell membrane by increasing its permeability and thus decreasing edema (Falconer et al., 1990; Hogan et al., 1982). Fluid will move out of tissue and be drained by the lymph system.

Precautions and Contraindications

When ultrasound is applied to older adults or others who have sensory impairment or decreased circulation, they should be monitored closely. If ultrasound is used directly over certain implants, heat may become focused on the surface of implants, resulting in burns. There is ongoing research being conducted on ultrasound application over fracture sites (Lee et al., 1990; Michlovitz, 1990).

Ultrasound should never be applied directly over the eyes, heart, pacemaker, testes, malignant tissue, tissues prone to hemorrhage, laminectomy, areas exposed to radiation therapy, infection, thrombophlebitis, or disc herniations. However, ultrasound can be applied to sites distant from these areas for pain relief (Lee et al., 1990; Michlovitz, 1990).

Reimbursement

Ultrasound therapy is reimbursed by almost all insurance agencies and the Center for Medicare and Medicaid Services.

Treatment Method

Ultrasound is energy in the form of acoustic vibration above audible range above 20,000 Hz (Perret et al., 2006). Sound waves are introduced into the body safely to achieve therapeutic effects. Therapeutic ultrasound is used at frequencies of .75–3 MHz at intensities of 0.1–2.0 W/cm². Therapeutic heating can be achieved in superficial structures or those up to 3–5 cm deep (Michlovitz, 1990) and may increase tissue temperatures by 39–41°F/4–5°C. One study indicated heating depths to 8 cm (O'Young, Young, & Stiens, 2002). The higher the collagen content of the tissue, the more ultrasound energy is absorbed. A study by Draper and colleagues (1995) identified specific treatment parameters by measuring temperature increases at multiple intensities at 1 MHz and 3 MHz frequencies.

A coupling agent is necessary for sound wave penetration through the skin to underlying structures. A water-based gel is most commonly used. Ultrasound can also be applied underwater in specific conditions. Phonophoresis is a method of introducing medication into the skin using ultrasound. This medication is usually a steroid compound mixed with gel. Insurance companies mandate a clinician's order for phonophoresis because it involves medication.

Ultrasound can be thermal or nonthermal (subsensory). The thermal effects of ultrasound are the same as for superficial heating and have been listed previously. Nonthermal effects include acoustic streaming and cavitation. Acoustic streaming is the movement of fluids along the cell membrane as a result of the sound waves, thereby decreasing subacute edema. Cavitation is the formation of air bubbles under the sound head that theoretically will change cell membrane permeability, also reducing edema.

The physical therapist or physical therapy assistant can modify several parameters of the ultrasound wave to produce desired effects. Modifications in frequency allow the therapist to target deep or superficial structures. Altering the duty cycle (percent output) and the intensity allows for thermal or nonthermal applications. There are a variety of sound-head sizes to allow for the treatment of small, large, or hard-to-reach areas. The angle of ultrasound application to the target tissue will affect outcomes. Eighty- to ninety-degree angles of application demonstrate the greatest thermal effects (Kimura, Gulick, Shelly, & Ziskin, 1998). Ultrasound can also be combined with electrical stimulation. The ultrasound head acts as an electrode to supply sound waves and electrical stimulation. No studies have demonstrated the effectiveness of this combination being superior to either modality applied separately (Lee et al., 1990). Therapeutic ultrasound is used frequently and has been proven to be effective.

Iontophoresis

Iontophoresis is commonly used to treat pain and inflammation in small, specific areas. The medication of choice is dexamethasone. Other compounds and their clinical uses include acetic acid to decrease calcium deposits such as those found in calcific tendonitis, lidocaine for soft tissue pain, citrate for rheumatoid arthritis, iodine for sclerotic scar tissue, magnesium as a muscle relaxant, and salicylate for pain relief and plantar warts (Li & Scudds, 1995).

Indications

Iontophoresis is indicated in the treatment of tendonitis, bursitis, trigger points, plantar fasciitis, costochondritis, small muscle spasms, capsulitis, and those conditions listed in the previous paragraph.

Precautions and Contraindications

It is not uncommon for the skin to develop a slight rash following iontophoresis. This is due to the direct current needed to deliver the medication, not to the medication itself. The skin must be intact, and patient sensitivity to the medication should be monitored prior to and following the therapy. Iontophoresis should never be used over the site of a pacemaker, an area of severe osteoarthritis, or over an acute injury with active bleeding. The therapy is also contraindicated if the patient has sensitivity to the medication.

Reimbursement

Insurance coverage is variable and needs to be confirmed prior to treatment. If an insurance carrier reimburses for iontophoresis, a physician's order is mandatory.

Iontophoresis Method

Iontophoresis is a process that uses direct current to propel medication across intact skin into underlying tissue. It is a noninvasive, usually painless, site-specific delivery of molecules for multiple clinical purposes. A phoresor has two polar opposite pads. If the medication has an overall positive polarity, it is placed under the positive pad. When the phoresor is activated, the positive current running through the pad will drive the positively charged molecules into the tissue. Studies have shown penetration up to 12 mm (Anderson, Morris, Boeh, Panus, & Sembrowich, 2003; Bolin & Goforth, 2004; Soroko, Repking, Clemment, Mitchell, & Berg, 2002). Iontophoresis has been used clinically for 50 years by dermatologists and physical therapists with no documented severe adverse reactions (Soroko et al., 2002).

The most common use of iontophoresis is to deliver dexamethasone, a synthetic glucocorticol steroid used for decreasing inflammation and pain to the painful site. The dose delivered is effective but extremely small. When compared to injection of similar medication, the risks of infection and systemic reactions are decreased. Iontophoresis delivers a greater concentration to a specific site than oral medication (Costello & Jeske, 1995; Nowicki, Hummer, Heidt, & Colosimo, 2002). Patients can receive iontophoresis utilizing dexamthasone concurrent with other steroid delivery therapies.

In the past, application was performed only in clinics and only lasted 10–20 minutes. Recently "take-home" patches have been developed that allow the treatment to occur throughout the day. The patches are very low profile and are worn from 4 to 24 hours depending on the manufacture and type. Preliminary reports find that patches worn for a longer time allow a greater amount of medication to be absorbed by the tissue and hence better outcomes. Others contend that the lower dose of medication when delivered over an extended time frame is flushed from the area before it can be effective.

Aqua Therapy

Aquatic (pool) therapy will promote relaxation, increase circulation, restore mobility, strengthen muscles, improve balance, increase proprioceptive input, and increase metabolic activity. Exercises can be performed with decreased weight-bearing stress on joints.

Indications

Aquatic therapy is prescribed for those with pain, joint stiffness, muscle weakness, osteoarthritis and rheumatoid arthritis, obesity, neurological disorders, joint replacements, polio, ankylosing spondolytis, osteoporosis, and others. Hydrotherapy provides a safe environment for guided exercises for the neurologically impaired.

Physiologic Effects

Elderly or other individuals with cardiovascular disease best tolerate water temperatures below 100.4°F/38°C (Michlovitz, 1990). There is an increase in venous return and systolic blood pressure (Allison, Maresh, & Armstrong, 1998). Cardiac output and stroke volume increase. Immersion to the neck will increase central blood volume by 60%, and cardiac volume increases nearly 30% (American College of Sports Medicine, 1995; Risch, Koubenec, Beckmann, Lange, & Gauer, 1987). Heart rate increases are less than with comparable land exercises and VO_2 max decreases (Butts, Tucker, & Greening, 1991; Butts, Tucker, & Smith, 1991).

Individuals with pulmonary diseases do best with water temperatures lower than 100.4°F/38°C. Expiratory reserve volume will decrease by 50% and vital capacity can decrease by 6–12% with immersion to the shoulders. This combination will increase the work of breathing by 60% (Hong, Cerretelli, Cruz, & Rahn, 1969; Perk, Perk, & Boden, 1996). It has been shown that hydrotherapy decreases the chance of exercise-induced asthma (Bar-Or & Inbar, 1992; Bar-Yishay, 1982).

Hydrostatic pressure resulting from immersion will increase urine output, and sodium and potassium production (Epstein, 1976). These effects will increase with the depth of immersion (Michlovitz, 1990).

Precautions and Contraindications

Individuals with decreased thermal sensation, infection, impaired cognition, recent skin grafts, alcohol use, fear of water, and urinary incontinence should be monitored closely. Individuals with poor strength, endurance, range of motion, or balance may require additional assistance. Individuals who use cardiac medication or medications that effect alertness should also be monitored closely.

Aquatic therapy should not be prescribed for those with maceration around a wound, active bleeding, cardiac instability, bowel incontinence, severe epilepsy, or suicide ideation. Individuals who have multiple sclerosis or have a decreased ability to thermal regulate should not utilize hot whirlpools or pool settings above the recommended standards.

Reimbursement

Many insurance companies will reimburse for aquatic therapy if it is under the direction of a physical therapist. Insurance carriers may also have specific guidelines for coverage and limits in duration of therapy.

Aquatherapy Methods

Pool therapy is performed in water that is waist to shoulder deep or in deep water using floats. Water temperature is generally 91–104°F/33–40°C (Allison et al., 1998; Cinder, Sunnerhagen, Schaufelberger, Schaufelberger, & Andersson, 2005; Michlovitz, 1990). Older adults who cannot tolerate the stress of land exercises can perform aerobic activities and strengthening and stretching exercises in water.

There are three major effects of exercise in water. The first is thermal effects that will increase tissue temperature and blood flow. Agitation provided by jets in the pool or whirlpool tank is the second effect. Agitation will decrease muscle spasms, joint pain, and stiffness. Exercises can be facilitated if performed in the direction of agitation flow or resisted if against the flow. The stimulation of skin receptors acts as a counterirritant to pain (Michlovitz, 1990). The third effect is buoyancy. Buoyancy provides reduced stress and compressive forces on weight-bearing joints, muscles, and soft tissue. Water will provide resistance or assistance to movement even without agitation. Circulation is improved and edema decreased.

Soft Tissue Mobilization

Soft tissue mobilizations (massage) will reduce pain, decrease muscle spasm, improve blood circulation, improve lymph drainage, decrease trigger point, decrease blood pressure (Moyer, Rounds, & Hannum, 2004), decrease heart rate (Moyer et al., 2004), and promote relaxation.

Indications

Soft tissue mobilizations are often applied to individuals with chronic pain (Griffin, 2003; Plews-Ogan, Owens, Goodman, Wolfe, & Schorling, 2005; Walach, Büthlin, & König, 2003), acute pain, edema, fibromyalgia, myofascial pain, muscle spasm, trigger point bands, pain related to cancer, headaches, arthritis, insomnia, reduced range of motion, depression, and anxiety (Walach, et al., 2003).

Physiologic Effects

Stimulation of muscle and fascial tissue results in muscle relaxation and improved flexibility (Lee et al., 1990). Scar tissue and connective tissue can be loosened by this method of therapy. A decreased cortisol blood level combined with increased levels of serotonin and dopamine act together to decrease stress (Field, Hernandez-Reif, Diago, Schanberg, & Kuhn, 2005) and pain. Sleep patterns have also shown to improve with soft tissue mobilization (Field, 2002).

Precautions and Contraindications

Soft tissue mobilizations are not entirely risk free. Injury is most often caused by a layperson or the utilization of other than standard techniques (Ernst, 2003). Soft tissue mobilizations should not be applied in the presence of certain forms of cancer, phlebitis, some cardiac problems, select skin conditions, and over a fracture site.

Reimbursement

Many insurance companies will not cover "massage" as applied by a physical therapist or by a certified massage therapist. However, "soft tissue mobilizations" when provided in the physical therapy setting are reimbursed. Several Worker's Compensation carriers will now reimburse massage provided by a certified massage therapist. This is much more cost-effective than having the same treatment provided by a physical therapist or physical therapist assistant.

Soft Tissue Mobilization Methods

Soft tissue mobilizations imply a clinical application of massage techniques to treat specific soft tissue disorders. There are many different techniques, and the nomenclature is often confusing. Recently a group of authors worked to create taxonomy to classify and standardize massage techniques. *Relaxation massage* is used to relax the body and promote wellness by moving body fluids, removing wastes, decreasing pain, and relaxing muscles. Techniques include petrissage (gliding), effleurage (kneading), friction massage, and others. *Clinical massage* focuses on treatment of muscle, fascia, and other body systems. Techniques include trigger point release, myofascial release, and others. *Movement re-education* uses assisted movement to enhance posture, movement, and body awareness. Common forms include Feldenkrais, muscle energy technique, and strain- counterstrain. The last category is *energy work,* which focuses on moving stagnant or blocked "energy" (Sherman, Dixon, Thompson, & Cherkin, 2006). The reader is referred to Chapter 8 for more detail related to this therapy. Most therapists use a combination of techniques to obtain therapeutic results. A cream or oil is commonly applied to the skin prior to soft tissue work. Not only does this decrease irritating friction on the skin, but some topical creams will also provide the sensation of cold or heat, which acts as a counter-irritant to pain (Griffin, 2003).

Soft tissue mobilizations may be applied with a sustained force or mobile force. The depth of the treatment is not only changed by increasing pressure, but can also be determined by the angle of force application. To reach deeper tissues, the force of massage application needs to be applied more perpendicular to the body part. Several techniques, such as trigger point release, may not be comfortable at the time of application, but the desired effect may still be pain relief. Frequently, depending on how restricted and congested the treated tissue is, there is an increase in pain for several hours following treatment. Patients are encouraged to drink plenty of noncaffeinated beverages to assist in flushing waste products from the treated tissue. Pain relief from tissue mobilization may last several hours to several days (Hasson, Arnetz, Jelveus, & Edelstam, 2004). There is often a concurrent decrease in medication use when tissue mobilization is effective.

Joint Mobilization

Indications

Joint mobilizations are used to decrease pain, improve joint range of motion, break scar tissue adhesions, improve joint nutrition, and promote joint healing Mobilizations may be applied to individuals who have chronic pain, painful joint(s), post-surgical scarring, loss of range of motion, and functional limitations.

Physiological Effects

Synovial fluid is found inside all joints and nourishes the joint surfaces. Movement is necessary to move the synovial fluid and bathe the joint surfaces. With aging, active joint movement and range of motion decreases, and hence joint health decreases. Mobilizations will improve joint function and health utilizing an external moving force to decrease restrictions in the joint capsule and supporting ligaments. Mobilizations may also calm the sympathetic nervous system, decreasing its output and resulting in fewer muscle spasms and less pain.

Precautions and Contraindications

Extreme care should be observed when mobilizing joints of the elderly, those with osteoporosis, severe osteoarthritis, rheumatoid arthritis, chronic pain, joint replacements, post-surgical sites, and individuals on chronic steroid use. Mobilizations should never be applied to an unstable joint, to an infected joint, or near a healing fracture.

Reimbursement

Joint mobilizations are reimbursed by most insurers under the category of "manual therapy."

Joint Mobilization Methods

All joints are composed of two articulating surfaces covered in cartilage. The joint capsule surrounds the joint and contains the synovial fluid to the inside of the joint. Over time or with injury, joint cartilage loses its ability to bind water and its fibers begin to fray. The capsule's fibers also change and become more fibrous and less elastic. These changes result in stiff, painful joints. Because joints are nourished by movement and the bathing of synovial fluid over the cartilage surfaces, any lack of motion further compromises the health of a joint. With aging, there is a loss of overall body mobility and a tendency toward joint dysfunction. Joints will compress in response to ligament tightness, capsule tightness, loss of hydration, and lack of movement. Overall, this results in increased pain and loss of function.

Joint mobilizations can be applied to any joint, from the large hip joints to the small facet joints of the spine. One bone is slid across the other, taking up the slack in the joint capsule. From there, gentle or aggressive force may be applied to stretch the capsule. Distracting joints, pulling the joint surfaces apart, will also improve range of motion.

Mobilizations can be applied to the joint for direct effects such as improving range of motion and decreasing pain, or for indirect effects. The indirect effects involve the sympathetic nervous system (SNS). The SNS lies along the spine at the levels of vertebrae T1 through L2. The ganglia, containing the cell bodies, lie very close to the spinous processes of these vertebrae. Gentle, oscillatory (low-grade and repetitive) mobilizations applied to the region of the SNS ganglia may assist in decreasing pain in remote sites by reducing sympathetic output from the ganglia.

Exercise

There are physiological changes that occur with aging that can contribute to chronic pain. Muscle tissue becomes stiffer and there is a decrease in muscle mass (Brooks & Faulkner, 1994; Lexell, 1995). This results in decreased strength, power, and endurance. There is an overall increase in connective tissue with a gradual decrease in tissue elasticity (Evans, 1999), resulting in a decrease in range of motion. There are fewer spinal cord neurons, which contributes to a decrease in nerve conduction velocity (Shock, 1967). There is an also increase in fat content of tissues. Exercise is an obvious solution to counteract these processes.

The American Geriatrics Society recommends a comprehensive program for treating persistent pain in the elderly population. The program should include pharmacology, education, behavior, and exercise. Studies have indicated that everyone, regardless of age, can benefit from exercise (Charette et al., 1991; Coggan et al., 1992; Fiatarone et al., 1994; Frontera, Meredith, O'Reilly, Knuttgen, & Evans, 1998; Mazzeo & Tanaka, 2001). Individuals in their nineties demonstrated significant improvements in muscle size and strength as well as in functional mobility (Fiatarone et al., 1990). Exercise will positively affect the chronically ill (Buchner, Beresford, Larson, LaCroix, & Wagner, 1992), often decreasing pain associated with many illnesses. Mortality is improved in all who exercise (Buchner et al., 1992; Paffenbarger, Hyde, Wing, & Hsieh, 1986; Paffenbargeret al., 1994). Individuals who have led a sedentary life but begin to exercise in later years will still benefit from exercise (Fiatarone et al., 1990). However, significant health protection and longevity are ensured if individuals are active throughout life (Blair, 1995). One study demonstrated that elderly men who were active for more than 20 years demonstrated reaction times faster than sedentary men in their twenties (Spirduso & Clifford, 1978).

The American College of Sports Medicine recommends stress testing prior to starting an exercise program for males over the age of 40 and females over the age of 50. There is a small risk of sudden death with heavy exertion, but the health benefits of regular exercise far outweigh this risk (Franklin, 1994; Mittleman, 1993). There is less risk of death with exercise if the individual has been active on a regular basis (Siscovick, Weiss, Fletcher, & Lasky, 1984). It is important to remember that strenuous exercise is not required to achieve positive effects.

In any structured exercise program, there should be a warm-up portion, the exercise modality, and then a cool-down. Paffenbarger and colleagues (1986) recommend that exercise should occur in moderation for 30 minutes, three to seven times per week. Three components should be included in all exercise regimes: strengthening, aerobic conditioning, and flexibility/balance (Nied & Franklin, 2002).

Decreased muscle strength is not only a result of a decrease in motor units and hence muscle mass, but of decreased daily muscle loading (Booth, 1994; Brooks & Faulkner, 1994). Progressive resistive exercises have been responsible for marked decreases in pain and improvement in functional mobility (Binder et al., 2002; Binder et al., 2005; Coleman, Buchner, Cress, Chan, & deLaterur, 1996). Patients with arthritis and joint symptoms demonstrate strength gains comparable to others without joint dysfunction. Other etiologies should be considered before attributing pain with exercise to arthritis. Exercise programs, specifically strengthening programs, cause discomfort as the musculoskeletal system is challenged.

Every comprehensive exercise plan needs an aerobic exercise component. Kohrt and colleagues (1998) found the heart rate method is effective when determining proper intensity for aerobic exercise. Interestingly, intense aerobic exercise does not provide any increased benefit than moderate exercise (Evans, 1999; Lamberg, 1998; Lee et al., 2001; Pate et al., 1995). The duration of exercise, not the intensity, determines functional gains.

Balance and flexibility are intimately intertwined, especially in the lower extremities. For example, a decreased range of motion through the ankle will result in a loss of proprioception. Loss of proprioception or loss of the ability of the brain to tell where the ankle is in space, combined with a lack of motion, results in a decrease in balance (Gajdosik, Vander Linden, McNair, Williams, & Riggin, 2005). Joint restrictions are not only a safety hazard but also are generally painful. Several other physiologic changes contribute to motion loss in any joint, but the greatest contributor is the loss of physical activity. Many studies have demonstrated improvements in balance and flexibility with a decrease in fear of falling (Lord, Caplan, & Ward, 1993; Lord et al., 2003; Liu-Ambrose, Khan, Eng, Lord, & McKay, 2004; Taggart, 2002), in the elderly and in those with chronic pain.

Outcomes

Success of any exercise program depends upon tailoring it to meet the needs of the individual. Many individuals fear movement will cause an increase in pain. Appropriate education is critical to assist older adults in overcoming this fear. Evaluation of financial status, equipment available, and the ability to travel will assist in designing a successful program. Many elderly people benefit from the social aspect of group exercise, because chronic pain is associated with social isolation and depression (Gibson et al., 1994). The availability and need of an external support system should be considered. Determining which activities the individual enjoys and is motivated to perform is important in compliance and benefit.

Precautions and Contraindications

Precautions to any exercise include hypertension, cardiomyopathies, valvular disease, complex ventricular ectopy, certain medications, prolonged inactivity, and cognition deficits (American College of Sports Medicine, 1998). Medical clearance for initiating an exercise program is essential.

Contraindications for exercise include recent electrocardiogram changes, myocardial infarction, unstable angina, uncontrolled hypertension, uncontrolled cardiac arrhythmia, third degree heart block, acute heart failure, and uncontrolled metabolic diseases (American College of Sports Medicine, 1998). If exercise is requested, specific guidelines should be provided by the requesting practitioner. Vital signs need to be monitored frequently.

Reimbursement

Most insurance companies cover exercise coded as "therapeutic exercise." Therapy visits to establish a home therapeutic exercise program are also covered.

Electrical Stimulation

Electrical stimulation (e-stim) is an extremely versatile modality. Electricity is a waveform that can be modified to produce various types of clinical electrical stimulation. The frequency, waveform, and intensity are parameters that are modified depending on treatment goals. TENS (Transcutaneous Electrical Nerve Stimulation), IFC (Interferential Current), and NMES (Neuromuscular Electrical Stimulation) are the most commonly used forms of e-stim for controlling chronic pain and muscle guarding/spasms.

Indications

Acute pain, chronic pain, phantom limb pain, postoperative pain, neurologic pain (Kosses, 2004), osteoarthritis, fibromyalgia, tendonitis, and bursitis have all responded favorably to electrical stimulation. Less common but effective uses include nausea control in patients on chemotherapy, regaining motor function following stroke, decreasing angina pectoris, decreasing urge incontinence (Kaye, 2005), decreasing joint contractions, and decreasing spasticity. Sympathetically mediated pain can also be decreased.

Physiologic Effects

Pain is relieved through several different avenues. The opiate-mediated control theory may be stimulated and the body will release its own natural painkillers, endorphins. Electrical stimulation may block pain signals to the brain via the pain gate control theory. Local blood flow is increased, which will promote healing, decrease edema, and flush pain mediators from the region. Local nerve stimulation will decrease pain. Muscle stimulation will induce relaxation.

Precautions and Contraindications

Electrodes should not be placed over the carotid arteries, or on the chest of individuals with cardiac disease. Electrodes should also not be placed over the eyes or over the head and neck in patients with epilepsy, neurologic disorder, or stroke. Individuals with impaired cognition, atrophic skin, open wounds, poor circulation, or poor sensation need constant monitoring during therapy. Stimulation should not occur over cancerous tissue (Kosses, 2004), in the mouth, or near the trigeminal nerve if there is a history of herpes zoster. E-stim over a spinal cord stimulator or interthecal pump should be performed only with extreme caution. Use of electrical stimulation on an extremity with an IV line should be monitored carefully as well. Electrical stimulation should not be used near demand-type pacemakers, over the carotid sinuses, or over a pregnant uterus.

Reimbursement

Electrical stimulation modalities performed in the clinic are billable. Currently, insurance reimbursement is easier to obtain for TENS and NMES home units than for IFC home units. There are many e-stim units available. Insurers may pay if the unit is provided through contracted suppliers. Some insurers reimburse for renting the units; others require purchase only.

Transcutaneous electrical nerve stimulator (TENS). TENS units have multiple settings for pain control. TENS stimulation can be at a subsensory level where the patient feels no stimulation; at the sensory level where the patient feels a buzzing or prickling sensation; at the motor level where a muscle contraction is elicited, and at a noxious level where the sensation is uncomfortable. Sensory-level or conventional TENS, which operates at 20–200 Hz, is most often used for pain control. Motor level can used for pain control but is not tolerated as well by patients. In general, frequencies used are from 60–80 Hz as they are more comfortable than lower frequencies. Asymmetric and biphasic waveforms are used to decrease skin irritation.

There are two major theories to explain how TENS controls pain (Kosses, 2004). The first is the pain-gate control theory, which states that small-diameter, slow-conducting nociceptive nerve fibers transmit painful stimuli to the spinal cord. TENS may diminish the sensation of pain by stimulating the faster sensory nerve fibers, blocking the sensation of pain to the spinal cord and hence the brain. The second theory is the opiate-mediated control theory. The naturally occurring endorphins and enkaphalins can be released with stimulation to the sensory nerves. The production of analgesia has various success rates, ranging from placebo to 95%, depending on the study (Braddom, 2002).

Many commercial TENS units offer multiple program settings so the patients can identify several that provide relief. The intensity of the stimulation is patient controlled and should never be painful with sensory-level and motor-level stimulation. The greatest factor to success with TENS use is pad/electrode placement (Kaye, 2005). The electrodes should surround the painful region. If this is ineffective, it has been suggested to apply the pads over acupuncture points (Roesch & Ulrich, 1980), involved nerve roots, along the course of a specifically involved peripheral nerve, on trigger points, or over the sympathetic ganglia. The patient may wear the unit for 10 minutes to 24 hours. Pain relief may start 20 to 60 minutes after the start of stimulation. Despite the precautions, TENS is highly acceptable and useful in the geriatric population for both acute and chronic conditions (Perret et al., 2006). Studies indicate a decrease in use of muscle relaxants, NSAIDS (nonsteroidal anti-inflammatory drugs), tranquilizers, steroids, opiate analgesics, and physical/occupational therapy services with transcutaneous electrical stimulation (Perret et al., 2006).

Interferential current (IFC). Interferential current is very similar to TENS stimulation. It is believed to penetrate deeper than TENS as it operates at higher frequencies (4,000–5,000 Hz). Because the skin offers less resistance at higher frequencies, some individuals may experience greater pain relief with IFC versus TENS. IFC is based on the summation of two alternating current signals of slightly different frequencies (Kaye, 2005). These currents must cross in the area being targeted for treatment to be effective. The parameters may then be adjusted to achieve sensory-level stimulation, motor-level stimulation, or both. A home IFC unit was recently introduced.

Neuromuscular electrical stimulation (NMES). Direct effects of neuromuscular electrical stimulation include decreased edema, reduced muscle fatigue, muscle strengthening, and improved range of motion. NMES also provides endurance training for deconditioned muscles and muscle re-education. Indirectly, pain will be relieved with these applications. Sequential stimulation has recently been introduced to combine the benefits of alternating current stimulation (IFC) and pulsed current or NMES. Sequential stimulations combine a period of pain-relieving stimulation followed by a period of muscle contraction. The muscle contractions will promote strengthening, decrease edema, and promote relaxation. Several easy-to-use home models are available.

SUMMARY

Physical therapists and assistants are valuable participants on health care teams managing elderly individuals with persistent pain. They are well educated and trained in multiple modalities to provide relief without medication, many which have been reviewed. However, the importance of each individual's active participation in their own care cannot be overemphasized. Rakel and Barr (2003) reported that the modality with the greatest support for pain management is therapeutic exercise. This chapter reviewed numerous therapies that can benefit older adults with various etiologies of persistent pain.

REFERENCES

Abramson, D. I., Chu, L. S., & Tucks, J. R. (1966). Effect of tissue temperatures and blood flow on motor nerve conduction velocity. *Journal of the American Medical Association, 198,* 1082–1088.

Allen, R. J. (2006). Physical agents used in the management of chronic pain by physical therapists. *Physical Medicine and Rehabilitation Clinics of North America, 17*(2), 315–345.

Allison, T. G., Maresh, C. M., & Armstrong, L. E. (1998). Cardiovascular responses in whirlpool bath at 40°C versus user-controlled temperatures. *Mayo Foundation of Medical Education and Research, 73*(3), 210–215.

American College of Sports Medicine. (1995). *Guidelines for exercise testing and prescription* (5th ed.). Baltimore: Williams and Wilkins.

American College of Sports Medicine Position Statement. (1998). Exercise and physical activity for older adults. *Medical Science in Sports and Exercise, 30,* 992–1008.

Anderson, C. R., Morris, R. L., Boeh, S. D., Panus, P. C., & Sembrowich, W. L. (2003). Effects on iontophoresis current magnitude and duration on dexamethasone deposition and localize drug retention. *Physical Therapy, 83,* 161–170.

Ansari, N. N., Egadi, S., Talebian, S., Naghdi, S., Mazaheri, H., Olyaei, G., et al. (2006). A randomized, single blind placebo controlled clinical trial on the effect of continuous ultrasound on low back pain. *Electromyographics and Clinical Neurophysiology, 46*(6), 329–336.

Baker, R. J., & Bell, G. W. (1991). The effect of therapeutic modalities on blood flow in the human calf. *Journal of Orthopedics and Sports Physical Therapy, 13,* 23–27.

Bar-Or, O., & Inbar, I. (1992). Swimming and asthma benefits and deleterious effects. *Sports Medicine, 14,* 397–405.

Bar-Yishay, E. (1982). Differences between swimming and running as stimuli for exercise-induced asthma. *European Journal of Applied Physiology, 48,* 387–397.

Binder, E. F., Schechtman, K. B., Ehsani, A. A., Steger-May, K., Brown, M., Sinacore, D. R., et al. (2002). Effects of exercise training on frailty in community-dwelling older adults: results of a randomized, controlled trial. *Journal of the American Geriatric Society, 50*(12), 1921–1928.

Binder, E. F., Yarasheski, K. E., Sterger-May, K., Sinacore, D. R., Brown, M., Schechtman, K. B., et al. (2005). Effects of progressive resistance training on body composition in frail older adults: Results of a randomized, controlled trial. *Journal of Gerontology, 60*(11), 1425–1431.

Blair, S. N. (1995). Physical fitness and all-cause mortality: A prospective study of healthy men and women. *Journal of the American Medical Association, 262,* 2395–2401.

Bolin, D., & Goforth, M. (2004). Electric delivery: Generally well tolerated by patients, iontophoresis has many uses for the rehab clinician. *Rehabilitation Management, 17*(10), 18–21.

Booth, F. W. (1994). Effect of aging on human skeletal muscle and motor function. *Medical Science in Sports and Exercise, 26,* 556–669.

Borrell, R. M., Parker, R., & Henley, R. J. (1980). Comparison of in-vivo temperatures produced by hydrotherapy, paraffin wax treatment and fluidotherapy. *Physical Therapy, 60*(10), 1272–1276.

Braddom, R. L. (2002). Physical agent modalities: Electrical stimulation. In R. L. Braddom (Ed.), *Physical medicine and rehabilitation* (2nd ed., pp. 440–487). Philadelphia: WB Saunders.

Brooks, S. V., & Faulkner, J. A. (1994). Skeletal muscle weakness in old age: Underlying mechanisms. *Medical Science in Sports and Exercise, 26*(4), 432–439.

Buchner, D. M., Beresford, S. A., Larson, E. B., LaCroix, A. Z., & Wagner, E. H. (1992). Effects of physical activity: Health status in older adults. II. Intervention studies. *Annual Review of Public Health, 13,* 469–488.

Butts, N. K., Tucker, M., & Greening, C. (1991). Physiologic responses to maximal treadmill and deep water running in men and women. *American Journal of Sports Medicine, 19,* 612–614.

Butts, N. K., Tucker, M., & Smith, R. (1991). Maximal responses to treadmill and deep water running in high school female cross country runners. *Research Quarterly in Exercise and Sports, 62,* 236–239.

Charette, S. L., McEvoy, L., Pyka, G., Snow-Harter, C., Guido, D., Wiswell, R. A., et al. (1991). Muscle hypertrophy response to resistance training in older women. *Journal of Applied Physiology, 70*(5), 1912–1916.

Cinder, A., Sunnerhagen, K. S., Schaufelberger, M., Schaufelberger, M., & Andersson, B. (2005). Cardiorespiratory effects of warm water immersion in elderly patients with chronic heart failure. *Clinical Physiology and Functional Imaging, 25*(6), 313–317.

Clark. R.S.J., Hellon, R. F., & Lind, A. R. (1958). Vascular reactions of the human forearm to cold. *Clinical Science, 17,* 165–173.

Cobbold, A. F., & Lewis, O. J. (1956). Blood flow to the knee joint of the dog: effects of heating, cooling and adrenaline. *Journal of Physiology, 132,* 379–383.

Coggan, A. R., Spina, R. J., King, D. S., Rogers, M. A., Brown, M., Nemath, P. M., et al. (1992). Skeletal muscle adaptations to endurance training in 60- to 70-yr-old men and women. *Journal of Applied Physiology, 72*(5), 1780–1786.

Coleman, E. A., Buchner, D. M., Cress, M. E., Chan, B. K., & deLaterur, B. J. (1996). The relationship of joint symptoms with exercise performance in older adults. *Journal of the American Geriatric Society, 44*(1), 14–21.

Collins, K., Storey, M., & Peterson, D. (1986). Perineal nerve palsy after cryotherapy. *American Journal of Sports Medicine, 14,* 105–111.

Conolly, W. B., Paltos, N., & Tooth, R. M. (1972). Cold therapy—an improved method. *Medical Journal of Australia, 2,* 42–45.

Costello, C. T., & Jeske, A. H. (1995). Iontophoresis: Application in transdermal medication delivery. *Physical Therapy, 75,* 554–563.

Currier, D. P., & Kramer, J. F. (1982). Sensory nerve conduction: heating effects of ultrasound and infrared. *Physiotherapy Canada, 34,* 241–251.

Draper, D. O., Casetl, J. C., & Castel, D. (1995). Rate of temperature increase in human muscle during 1 MHz and 3 MHz continuous ultrasound. *Journal of Orthopedics and Sports Physical Therapy, 22*(4), 142–150.

Edwards, H. E., et al. (1978). Effects of temperature on muscle energy metabolism and endurance during successive isometric contractions, sustained to fatigue, of the quadriceps muscle in man. *Journal of Physiology, 220,* 335.

Epstein, M. (1976). Cardiovascular and renal effects of head-out water immersion in man. *Circulation Research, 39*(5), 620–628.

Ernst, E. (2003). The safety of massage. *Rheumatology, 42*(9), 1101–1106.

Evans, W. J. (1999). Exercise training guidelines for the elderly. *Medicine and Science in Sports and Exercise, 31*(1), 12–17.

Falconer, J., Hayes, K. W., & Chang, R. W. (1990). Therapeutic ultrasound in the treatment of musculoskeletal conditions. *Arthritis Care Research, 3*(2), 85.

Fiatarone, M. A., Marks, E. D., Ryan, N. D., Meridith, C. N., Litsitz, L. A., & Evans, W. J. (1990). High-intensity strength training in nonagenarians: Effects on skeletal muscle. *Journal of the American Medical Association, 263*(22), 3029–3034.

Fiatarone, M. A., O'Neill, E. F., Ryan, N. D., Clements, K. M., Solares, G. R., Nelson, M. E., et al. (1994). Exercise training and nutritional supplementation for the physical frailty in very elderly people. *New England Journal of Medicine, 330,* 1976–1982.

Field, T. M. (2002). Massage therapy. *Medical Clinics of North America, 86*(1), 163–171.

Field, T., Hernandez-Reif, M., Diago, M., Schanberg, S., & Kuhn, C. (2005). Cortisol decreases and serotonin and dopamine increases following massage therapy. *International Journal of Neurosciences, 115*(10), 1397–1413.

Fox, R. H., & Wyatt, H. T. (1962). Cold-induced vasodilatation in various areas of the body surface in man. *Journal of Physiology, 162,* 289–298.

Franklin, B. A. (1994). Exercise and cardiac complications: Do the benefits outweigh the risks? *Physician and Sportsmedicine, 22*(2), 56.

Freitas, L. S., Freitas, T. P., Silveira, P. C., Rocha, L. G., Pinho, R. A., & Streck, E. L. (2006). Effect of therapeutic pulsed ultrasound on parameters of oxidative stress in skeletal muscle after injury. *Cell Biology International, 31,* 482–488.

Frontera, W. R., Meredith, C. N., O'Reilly, K. P., Knuttgen, H. G., & Evans, W. J. (1998). Strength conditioning in older men: Skeletal muscle hypertrophy and improved function. *Journal of Applied Physiology, 64,* 1038–1044.

Gajdosik, R. L., Vander Linden, D. W., McNair, P. J., Williams, A. K., & Riggin, T. J. (2005). Effects of an eight week stretching program on the passive-elastic properties and function of the calf muscle in older women. *Clinical Biomechanics, 20,* 973–983.

Gibson, S. J., Katz, B., Corran, T. M., Farrell, M. J., & Helme, R. D. (1994). Pain in older persons. *Disability and Rehabilitation, 16*(3), 127–139.

Gloth, M. J., & Matesi, A. M. (2001a). Pain management in the elderly: Physical therapy and exercise in pain management. *Clinics in Geriatric Medicine, 17*(3), 9–18.

Gloth, M. J., & Matesi, A. M. (2001b). Physical therapy and exercise in pain management. *Clinics in Geriatric Medicine, 17*(3), 1–7.

Griffin, B. L. (2003). Massage therapy has a role in pain management. *Practical Pain Management.* Retrieved December 31, 2007, from http://www.amtamassage.org/news/painmanagement.html. Halle, J. S., Scoville, C. R., & Greathouse, D. G. (1981). Ultrasound's effect on the conduction latency of the superficial radial nerve in man. *Physical Therapy, 61,* 345–354.

Harkins, S. W., Price, D. D., & Martelli, M. (1986). Effects of age on pain perception: thermonociception. *Journal of Gerontology, 41*(1), 58–63.

Hartvikksen, K. (1962). Ice therapy in spasticity. *Acta Neurologica Scandinavica, 38,* 79–87.

Hasson, D., Arnetz, B., Jelveus, L., & Edelstam, B. (2004). A randomized clinical trial of the treatment effects of massage compared to relaxation tape recordings on diffuse long-term pain. *Psychotherapy and Psychosomatics, 73*(1), 17–24.

Herrick, R. T., & Herrick, S. (1992). Fluidotherapy clinical applications and techniques. *The Journal of MASA, 61*(12), 20–25.

Hogan, R. D., Burke, K. M., & Granklin, T. D. (1982). The effect of ultrasound on microvascular hemodynamics in skeletal muscle: effects during ischemia. *Microvascular Research, 23,* 370–381.

Hong, S. K., Cerretelli, R., Cruz, J. C., & Rahn, H. (1969). Mechanics of respiration during submersion in water. *Journal of Applied Physiology, 27*(4), 535–536.

Kaye, V. (2005). Transcutaneous electrical nerve stimulation. *Emedicine.* Retrieved December 31, 2007, from http://www.emedicine.com/pmr/topic26.htm.

Kimura, I. F., Gulick, D. T., Shelly, J., & Ziskin, M. C. (1998). Effects of two ultrasound devices and angles of application of the temperature of two tissue phantom. *Journal of Orthopedics and Sports Physical Therapy, 27*(1), 27–31.

Kohrt, W. M., Spina, R. J., Hoolszy, J. O., & Ehsani, A. A. (1998). Prescribing exercise in tensity for older women. *Journal of the American Geriatric Society, 46*(2), 129–133.

Kosses, R. (2004). Two types of E-stim. *Rehabilitation Management, 17*(7), 18, 20–21, 42.

Kramer, J. F. (1984). Ultrasound: Evaluation of its mechanical and thermal effects. *Archives of Physical Medicine and Rehabilitation, 65*(5), 223–227.

Lamberg, L. (1998). New guidelines on managing chronic pain in older persons. *Journal of the American Medical Association, 280*(4), 311–312.

LeBan, M. M. (1962). Collagen tissue: Implications of its response to stress in-vitro. *Archives of Physical Medicine and Rehabilitation, 43,* 461–469.

Lee, J. M., Rexrode, K. M., Cook, N. R., Hennekines, C. H., & Burin, J. E. (2001). Physical activity and coronary heart disease in women: Is "no pain, no gain" passé? *Journal of the American Medical Association, 285*(11), 1447–1454.

Lee, J. M., Warren, M. P., & Mason, S. M. (1978). Effects of ice on nerve conduction velocity. *Physiotherapy, 64,* 2–10.

Lee, M., Itoh, M., Yany, G., & Eason, A. (1990). The management of pain. In J. Loeser, Chapman, & W. Fordyce (Eds.), *Physical therapy and rehabilitation medicine* (pp. 1769–1788). Philadephia: Lea & Febiger.

Lehmann, J. D., Brunner, G. D., & Stow, R. W. (1958). Pain threshold measurements after therapeutic application of ultrasound, microwaves and infrared. *Archives of Physical Medicine and Rehabilitation, 39,* 560–578.

Lexell, J. (1995). Human aging, muscle mass, and fiber type composition. *Journal of Gerontology, 50A,* 11–16.

Li, L. C., & Scudds, R. A. (1995). Iontophoresis: an overview of the mechanisms and clinical application. *Arthritis Care and Research, 8*(1), 51–61.

Liu-Ambrose, T. Y., Khan, K. M., Eng, J. J., Lord, S. R., & McKay, H. A. (2004). Balance confidence improves with resistance or agility training: Increase is not correlated with objective change in fall risk and physical abilities. *Gerontology, 50,* 373–382.

Lord, S. R., Caplan, G. A., & Ward, J. A. (1993). Balance, reaction time, muscle strength in exercising and nonexercising older women: A pilot study. *Archives of Physical Medicine and Rehabilitation, 74,* 837–839.

Lord, S. R., Castell, S., Corcoran, J., Dayhew, J., Matters, B., Shan, A., et al. (2003). The effects of group exercise on physical functioning and falls in frail older people living in retirement villages: A randomized, controlled trial. *Journal of the American Geriatric Society, 51*(12), 1685–1692.

Major, T. C., Schwinghamer, J. M., & Winston, S. (1981). Cutaneous and skeletal muscle vascular responses to hypothermia. *American Journal of Physiology, 240*(6), 868–873.

Matsen, F. A., Questd, K., & Matsen, A. L. (1975). The effect of local cooling on post fracture healing. *Clinical Orthopedics, 109,* 201–209.

Mazzeo, R. S., & Tanaka, H. (2001). Exercise prescription of the elderly: Current recommendations. *Sports Medicine, 31*(11), 809–818.

McCarberg, B., & O'Connor, A. (2004). A new look at heat treatment for pain disorders. Part 1. *American Pain Society Bulletin, 14*(6). Retrieved January 3, 2008, from http://www.ampainsoc.org/pub/bulletin/nov04/inno1.htm.

Mense, S. (1978). Effects of temperature on the discharge of muscle spindles and tendon organs. *Pfleugers Archives, 374,* 159–168.

Michlovitz, S. L. (1990). *Thermal agents in rehabilitation* (3rd ed.). Philadelphia: FA Davis.

Middaugh, S. J., Levin, R. B., Kee, W. G., & Barchiesi, F. D. (1988). Chronic pain: It's treatment in geriatric and younger patients. *Archives in Physical Medicine and Rehabilitation, 69,* 1021–1026.

Mittleman, M. A. (1993). Triggering of acute myocardial infarction by heavy physical exertion. *New England Journal of Medicine, 329,* 1677–1685.

Moore, J. H., Gieck, J. H., Saliba, E. N., Perrin, D. H., Ball, D. W., & McCue, F. C. (2000). The biophysical effects of ultrasound on median nerve distal latencies. *Electromyographic Clinics of Neurophysiology, 40*(3), 169–180.

Moyer, C. A., Rounds, J., & Hannum, J. W. (2004). A meta-analysis of massage therapy research. *Psychological Bulletin, 130*(1), 3–18.

Nied, R. J., & Franklin, B. (2002). Promoting and prescribing exercise for the elderly. *American Family Physician, 65*(3), 1–12.

Nobel, J. G., Lee, V., & Griffin-Nobel, F. (2007). Therapeutic ultrasound: The effects upon cutaneous blood flow in humans. *Ultrasound Medical Biology, 33*(2), 278–285.

Nowicki, D., Hummer, C. D., Heidt, R. S., & Colosimo, A. J. (2002). Effects of iontophoresis versus injection administration of dexamethasone. *American College of Sports Medicine, 34*(8), 1294–1301.

O'Connor, A., & McCarberg, B. (2005). A new look at heat treatment of pain disorders, part 2. *American Pain Society Bulletin, 15*(1). Retrieved January 3, 2008, from http://www.ampainsoc.org/pub/bulletin/win05/inno1.htm.

O'Young, B. J., Young, M. A., & Stiens, S. A. (2002). *Physical medicine and rehabilitation secrets* (2nd ed.). Philadelphia: Hanley & Belfus.

Paffenbarger, R. S., Kampert, J. B., Lee, I. M., Hyde, R. T., Leung, R. W., & Wing, A. L. (1994). Changes in physical activity and other lifeway patterns influencing longevity. *Medical Science in Sports and Exercise, 26,* 857–863.

Paffenbarger, R. S., Hyde, R. T., Wing, A. L., & Hsieh, C. C. (1986). Physical activity, all-cause mortality and longevity of college alumni. *New England Journal of Medicine, 314,* 605–613.

Pate, R. R., Pratt, M., Blair, S. M., Haskell, W. L., Macera, C. A., Bouchard, C., et al. (1995). Physical activity and public health: Recommendation from the Centers of Disease Control and Prevention and the American College of Sports Medicine. *Journal of the American Medical Association, 266,* 1535–1542.

Payne, C. (1984). Ultrasound for post-herpatic neuralgia. *Physiotherapy, 70,* 96–102.

Perk, J., Perk, L., & Boden, C. (1996). Adaptation of COPD patients to physical training on land and in water. *European Respiratory Journal, 9*(2), 248–252.

Perkins, J., Li, M. C., & Nicholas, C. H. (1950). Cooling as a stimulus to smooth muscle. *American Journal of Physiology, 163,* 14–26.

Perret, D. M., Rim, J., & Cristan, A. (2006). A geriatrician's guide to the use of physical modalities in the treatment of pain and dysfunction. *Clinics in Geriatric Medicine, 22*(2), 331–353.

Plews-Ogan, M., Owens, J. E., Goodman, M., Wolfe, P., & Schorling, J. (2005). A pilot study evaluation: mindfulness-based stress reduction and massage for the management of chronic pain. *Journal of Geriatric Internal Medicine, 20*(12), 1136–1138.

Rakel, B., & Barr, J. O. (2003). Physical modalities in chronic pain management. *Nursing Clinics of North America, 38*(3), 477–494.

Risch, W. E., Koubenec, H. J., Beckmann, U., Lange, S., & Gauer, O. H. (1987). The effect of graded immersion on heart volume, central venous pressure, pulmonary blood distribution and heart rate in man. *Pfleugers Archives: European Journal of Physiology, 374,* 115–118.

Robertson, V. J. (2002). Dosage and treatment response in randomized clinical trials of therapeutic ultrasound. *Physical Therapy in Sports, 3,* 124–133.

Roesch, R., & Ulrich, D. E. (1980). Physical therapy management in the treatment of chronic pain. *Physical Therapy, 60*(1), 53–57.

Sherman, K. J., Dixon, M. W., Thompson, D., & Cherkin, D. C. (2006). Development of a taxonomy to describe massage treatments for musculoskeletal pain. *BMC Complementary Alternative Medicine, 6,* 24.

Shock, N. W. (1967). Physical activity and the rate of aging. *Canadian Medical Association Journal, 96,* 836–838.

Siscovick, D. S., Weiss, N. S., Fletcher, R. H., & Lasky, T. (1984). The incidence of primary cardiac arrest during vigorous exercise. *New England Journal of Medicine, 311,* 874–879.

Soroko, M. C., Repking, M. C., Clemment, J. A., Mitchell, P. L., & Berg, L. (2002). Treatment of plantar verrucae using 2% sodium salicylate iontophoresis. *Physical Therapy, 82,* 1184–1191.

Spirduso, W. W., & Clifford, P. (1978). Replication of age and physical activity effects on reaction and movement time. *Journal of Gerontology, 33,* 26–33.

Taggart, H. M. (2002). Effects of Tai Chi exercise on balance, functional mobility, and fear of falling among older women. *Applied Nursing Research, 15*(4), 235–242.

Trudel, D., Duley, J., Zastrow, I., Kerr, E. W., Davidson, R., & McDermid, J. C. (2004). Rehabilitation for patients with lateral epicondylitis: A systematic review. *Journal of Hand Therapy, 17*(2), 243–266.

Wadsworth, H., & Chanmugam, A. P. (1988). Electrophysical agents in Physiotherapy (2nd ed.). Marrickville: Science Press.

Walach, H., Büthlin, C., & König, M. (2003). Efficacy of massage therapy in chronic pain: A pragmatic randomized trial. *Alternative and Complementary Medicine, 9*(6), 837–846.

Wright, V., & Johns, R. J. (1961). Quantitative and qualitative analysis of joint stiffness in normal subjects and in patients with connective tissue diseases. *American Rheumatology Disease, 20,* 36–43.

CHAPTER 8

Mind-Body and Energy Therapies

Susan D. Eckes Peck and Amanda Gentili

Therapies providing relaxation and balance of the energy field are an integral part of providing holistic care in the treatment of persistent pain in elders. Many clients eliminate or reduce the number of medications taken to relieve persistent pain when such therapies are used. Pain relief leads to improved quality of life and participation in society.

Current research, supported through the National Institutes of Health (NIH), National Center for Complementary and Alternative Medicine (NCCAM), and national professional health care organizations, provides evidence of multiple methods of relieving pain without medications or in addition to them. The NCCAM has increased research funding of therapies since 1992 from $2 million annually to $122 million this past year. Research funded primarily supports use of complementary therapies (http://nccam.nih.gov/news/camsurvey_fs1. htm). Therapies such as distraction, relaxation techniques, guided imagery or hypnotherapy, biofeedback, energy techniques, massage, and acupuncture are among numerous techniques under investigation to help relieve pain.

The World Health Organization (WHO) supports the use of safe and effective complementary therapies and the dissemination of information about them to consumers. Guidelines released June 22, 2004 encourage the development of "context specific and reliable information for consumer use of alternative medicines" (World Health Organization, 2006). Such information assists consumers to select appropriate therapies, such as mind-body and energy therapies, from reputable practitioners.

The Older Americans Act (OAA) "embodies our nation's compassion toward ensuring the dignity and independence of our older citizens by promoting older Americans' full participation in society, and supporting their overwhelming desire to remain living in their own homes and communities for as long as possible" (Older Americans Act, 2006). Relief of pain in elders, using mind-body and energy techniques that relax and balance the energy field, facilitates achievement of the OAA, WHO, and NCCAM goals.

Americans have been using complementary therapies for many years (Bodane & Brownson, 2002; Eisenberg, Davis, Ettner, Appel, Wilkey, et al., 1998). The most common uses of therapies are for chronic illnesses, including pain relief. People choose complementary therapies because therapists include them more fully in their care, and treatments eliminate (in some cases) or reduce medication therapy. The public pays more out of pocket on complementary therapies than they pay out of pocket for Western medical model health care (Eisenberg et al., 1998). Health professionals frequently note that clients make choices about prescribed medications and procedures, not always following advice as given. Given a client's openness to try therapies outside the mainstream, there is likely to be greater compliance with prescriptive recommendations if the provider works with the client's interests. At times, limitations to utilizing complementary therapies are reimbursement-related and not based on personal preference. Information cited in this chapter facilitates the provider guiding the client to make wise decisions.

Therapies discussed in this chapter are included in the practice of holistic nursing and are categorized by NCCAM as mind-body and energy therapies (http://nccam.nih.gov). The general technique of select mind-body therapies, relaxation, guided imagery, and hypnotherapy, and the energy therapies of healing touch and therapeutic touch are reviewed. The evidence base supporting use of the techniques for pain relief, and where to learn them or find a reputable practitioner, are discussed. Therapies are related to their role in relieving the pain-tension-anxiety cycle.

Pain is frequently accompanied by emotions and physical behaviors that can worsen pain. Affective components of persistent pain are feelings and emotions. The person may feel anger, depression, and anxiety regarding the lack of control of their pain and losses in role functions and leisure activity. The unknown meaning of the pain and its ramifications on one's life are cognitive stressors dealt with in addition to the pain itself. Emotional stress triggers sympathetic nervous system output, releasing norepinephrine. Fear of upcoming tests, of the next treatment, or of the unknown may also trigger release of norepinephrine. Norepinephrine release in turn increases the level of pain.

Pain affects posture and motion of the physical structure of the body. Muscles tighten, protecting affected areas, but cause further tension in the area as well. Protective muscle tension leads to strain and abnormal movement of contralateral limbs and muscles and may increase the areas of pain dealt with by the client. Anger may lead to muscles held in stiff resistance. Release of the anger may involve tightening of muscle groups to provide tension relief. Adaptive aides contribute to use of muscle groups beyond those usually involved with motions, causing muscle soreness, stiffness, and strain on groups of muscles not typically used for similar movement.

These affective, behavioral, and cognitive components of pain create a vicious cycle. The worse the pain, the worse the tension and anxiety. The more tension and anxiety present, the worse the pain. The cycle can be never-ending and can counter efficacy of traditional pain management therapies. Breaking the pain-tension-anxiety cycle using therapies that create the relaxation response may relieve pain alone; it can also increase efficacy of pain relief techniques and medications typically used in the allopathic system (Kazanowski & Laccetti, 2002).

Research evidence exists to provide scientific foundations for use of mind-body and energy techniques in the relief of pain. Research included focuses primarily on relief of pain and anxiety. Functional ability, sleep, and well-being are associated with pain, and as such are included.

Arguments exist regarding soundness of scientific method in studies of complementary therapies. The dilemma, though, is that performing the exact same treatment on every client may not be what is needed. For example, to perform the exact same hand movements on every client during an energy therapy may create a problem. In real practice, practitioners would evaluate the client's energy field and tailor the treatment to the client's needs. Using the same sequence of steps in treatments may not be what is needed by the client. An analogy would be using the same drug for every client who came into the medical system with an expressed symptom; if the symptom was not further explored, harm might be induced by the treatment. For example, if every client with a cough was given cough medication and no further assessment was done, heart failure, pneumonia, and lung cancer might be missed.

The world of complementary and alternative medicine (CAM) therapies is different and does not necessarily fit the Western scientific method of research well in every instance. Yet despite these concerns, the outcomes show positive effect with minimal detriment across complementary therapies. Outcomes need to be tracked to build the knowledge base and guide future research.

THERAPY OVERVIEWS

Mind-Body Therapies Creating the Relaxation Response

Mind-Body therapies creating the relaxation response provide basic, no-equipment-necessary means of breaking the pain-tension-anxiety cycle. Relaxation is fundamental to facilitation of all pain relief measures, including medications. Relaxation techniques used for a variety of physical (incisional pain, traumatic injuries, burns) causes of pain and related functional symptoms (altered mobility, activity intolerance, impaired sleep) relieve pain effectively.

Relaxation

Relaxation techniques range from breath work to tightening muscles and releasing the tension. Relaxation techniques are plentiful in the literature and on the Worldwide Web and are developed and supported by internationally renowned authors. Table 8.1 lists prominent relaxation experts and their Web sites. Web sites such as these can be used to find relaxation protocols for use in general and specific situations. Examples of relaxation protocols (breathing technique and progressive muscle relaxation) are found in Appendices A and B.

Practice of relaxation techniques creates the relaxation response, a physiologic condition opposite the stress response. The relaxation response is accompanied by the following physiologic changes: eased breathing, relaxed muscles, visualization of color in the mind's eye, slower, deeper breaths that become more shallow as relaxation deepens, more audible breathing, fluttering of eyelids and/or closing of eyes, blanching of skin around nose and mouth, toes pointing outward (supine), complete lack of muscle holding, dropping forward, backward, or sideways of head, and dropping of the shoulders (Achterberg, Dossey, & Kolkmeier, 1994). Presence of these physiologic changes provides evidence that relaxation occurred. The relaxation response facilitates blood flow and

TABLE 8.1   Relaxation Experts and Their Web Sites

Andrew Weil, MD (http://wwwldrweil.com/drw/ecs/index.html)	Bellaruth Naparstek (http://www.healthjourneys.com/)
Larry Dossey, MD (http://www.dosseydossey.com/larry/default.html)	Barbara Dossey, PhD, RN (http://www.dosseydossey.com/barbara/default.html)
Jeanne Achterberg, MD (http://www.jeanneachterberg.com)	Deepak Chopra, MD (http://www.chopra.com/3.html)

decreases tension in muscles throughout the body. Tension release provides relaxation of muscles and calms anxiety, thus reducing pain.

Guided Imagery

Nothing exists in our experience without an accompanying image. Images accompany emotions and precede every voluntary behavior. When receiving a diagnosis, clients form an image. The image in turn affects health outcomes. Some would argue that imagining a person, substance, or event causing healing is only placebo. Yet if placebo creates effect 30%–70% of the time, that's a significant outcome (Freeman, 2004).

Images occurring with traumatic events are saved by the brain, along with memory of the event itself. Triggers of images simultaneously recall the event. When the event is traumatic or somehow attached to the pain, image recall or seeing similar images will trigger the pain (Achterberg, 1985; Achterberg et al., 1994). Guided imagery and hypnotherapy facilitate change of the stored image to decrease pain.

Guided imagery and hypnotherapy are terms used to describe methods to facilitate the mind's imaging function without pain. Guided imagery is a thought process that invokes and uses the senses, including vision, sound, smell, taste, movement, positioning, touch, and intuition (Achterberg et al., 1994). Hypnosis is a state of attentive, focused concentration with suspension of some peripheral awareness. Components of the hypnotic state include absorption, alteration of attention, dissociation, and suggestibility (Freeman, 2001). Most people describe situations in which the mind wanders to a place they would rather be, a picture of the story they are reading or listening to, their favorite vacation spot, or a favorite time in their life. Guided imagery and hypnotherapy facilitate the person's imaging of those times or places, replacing the image of pain carried with them. Replacing the painful image with one of delight, fondness, or enjoyment breaks the pain-tension-anxiety cycle.

Guided imagery and hypnotherapy begin with relaxation, typically breath work or muscle softening as described earlier under the discussion on relaxation. Once breathing is focused and slowed, imagining function without pain or a favorite time or place begins. Use of the six senses (sight, smell, taste, touch—both physical and emotional, hearing, and intuition) assists imaging where and how the person would ideally be. The person is directed to see what is around them, where they are, what is above, below, in front of, behind them—in color, texture, motion, temperature, and other ways we "see." Images of the smells involved with the place or time are brought in. Examples may include crispness of the fall air, warm wafts of baking cookies, and the hint of fish scent in the ocean's gentle waves. Sounds involved in the place or time recreate the swish of the horse's tale, breezes through colored fall leaves, calls of birds flying overhead, or voices of companions. Tastes of the food or beverage consumed in the favorite place/time or the palated bite of the favorite wine drunk on the occasion may assist the person to create an image of function without pain or a favorite time or place. Touch is twofold; first, what is felt physically, and second, what is felt intuitively or emotionally with remembrance of the image, place, or functioning in comfort. Examples include feeling the particular garment or shoes worn in the place/time, the feel of the sand while walking on the beach, the coolness of the breeze gently wafting through the hair, the melt of muscles soaking in the hot tub, or the texture of the food or drink in the mouth. Intuitively, emotions or insights that come forth to remember the place/time create an "ah-ha," a stimulating vision of what to do next or how to respond to the situation.

Multiple types of imagery may be utilized. Cellular imagery works at the biologic level, changing perception of the structure or function of cells. Physiologic imagery creates pictures of normal, comfortable function of a body system or area. Psychological imagery maintains or brings about positive emotional states such as resiliency. Relationship imagery heals personal associations with others (Freeman, 2004).

Clinical use of imagery facilitates diagnosis when used by an intuitive healer (Myss, 2006) or the individual themselves. Diagnostic imagery assists definition of causes and physiologic connection/alterations within the body. Mental rehearsal imagery guides clients through what to expect and attainment of outcomes. An excellent example of mental rehearsal imagery is the text, *Prepare for Surgery, Heal Faster: A Guide of Mind-Body Techniques* by Huddleston (1996). Clients are guided through visioning the procedure to be done and its coveted end point. The coveted end point, end-state imagery, occurs with the use of mental rehearsal. Clinical practice of these techniques in my practice resulted in women with extensive vaginal repair surgeries voiding post-op one day after catheter removal, easing labor and birthing, surgical debridement procedures (burn wounds, infected chest wounds) done with no pain medication while the client rested in comfort, and increased range of motion following surgery to joints. Freeman (2004) describes vision quests as another means to provide information for individualized/meaningful imagery as clients search for meaning and purpose of the pain they experience. Clients work with a traditional cultural healer when performing vision quest.

Thorough assessment of the pain, its meaning for the person and effects of the pain on life, described by feelings, in sensory and emotional terms, provides information used to rehearse mental images. Verbal descriptions and drawings facilitate data collection. Drawings need not be artist quality, just personal representations of the client's vision of the pain. Interpretation of the drawing is the client's, not the practitioner's. Asking the client to describe the meaning of the color, shape, or size of the drawing, why certain pieces were included and why others were omitted helps the client to interpret their own drawing. Facilitating "finding meaning" assists clients to change the image they have of the pain and its cause (Borneman & Browne-Salzman, 2006).

Once the "painful" assessment is made, the client constructs a second image, in sensory and emotional terms as well as physical, of life in comfort. The comfort image (drawn or described) becomes the focus of the imagery used with the client. Positive outcomes become the focus of mental rehearsal imagery used for procedural testing or treatment. As an example, a client with a cancerous tumor in the throat drew the tumor and we discussed the effects it had on his life. In his second drawing, the tumor was replaced by healthy tissue and connected with positive changes in his life that he set out to create.

Another imagery/hypnotherapy format guides the person to visualize the pain leaving the body or being resolved. The person draws or forms mental pictures representing the essence of the pain or its origin and a second set of drawings or pictures depicting the essence of the body/mind/spirit without any pain. The drawing of being healed may be the only drawing necessary or preferred by the individual. Still other drawings depict resolution of the origin of pain—without the originating problem, the pain is gone.

Evidence of Efficacy for Pain Relief-Relaxation and Guided Imagery/Hypnotherapy

Relaxation and guided imagery techniques allow clients to retain a sense of control over their pain in addition to improving surgical outcomes, enhancing immune function, and prolonging life in clients with cancer (Tusek, Church, Strong, Grass, & Fazio, 1997). Experiences attained using relaxation and guided imagery techniques vary between clients, but overall there has been a very positive client response. Guided imagery is effective in producing clinically significant reductions in the experience of pain and noxious sensations (Sloman, 1995). With guided imagery clients are encouraged to confront and work through their feelings, fostering relaxation and a state of focused concentration. A sense of physical and emotional well-being is produced, enhancing the client's psychological and physiological wellness (Tusek et al., 1997).

Several studies have been conducted on the effects of relaxation and guided imagery on pain (Edgar, 1999; Tusek et al., 1997; Sloman, 1995; Stephens, 1999). Most studies conducted included elders, but studies related to elders alone are lacking. From cardiac care to conventional colorectal resections, research studies determined that relaxation and guided imagery are extremely helpful in the relief of pain from a number of conditions. Sloman (1995) showed that 67 subjects in the intermediate or advanced stages of cancer, randomly placed into progressive muscle relaxation and guided imagery groups, experienced significant reductions in nonopioid analgesia, present pain intensity, and overall pain severity. The simplicity of the techniques also makes them desired in situations with pain.

Astin (2004) conducted a meta-analysis of 25 randomized trials of varying mind-body therapies, including relaxation and guided imagery for varying pain conditions. Relaxation therapy combined with cognitive therapy, stress management, and coping skills training was found helpful for chronic low back pain. Relaxation and biofeedback therapy decreased tension and migraine headaches. Imagery, hypnosis, and relaxation improved recovery time and decreased postoperative pain, and mind-body approaches alleviated pain associated with invasive procedures.

The United States Agency for Health Care Policy and Research evaluated strength of evidence for relaxation effects of pain control. Findings showed strongly effective outcomes of reduced pain in a variety of medical conditions (Freeman, 2004). Relaxation and guided imagery, and relaxation and guided imagery with biofeedback, were useful to decrease pain and anxiety during wound debridement and dressing changes in burn victims. Anxiety, pain, cold, and shivering after tub treatments were reduced after being rehearsed in a state of deep calm (Achterberg et al., 1988).

Peck (1998) and Gordon and colleagues (1998) examined the use of progressive muscle relaxation and therapeutic touch for pain reduction in elders with arthritis. Subjects in both studies had reduced pain, improved functional ability, improved sleep, and enhanced well-being.

The work of Masaru Emoto has been instrumental to show the effects of positive imagery, thinking, and verbalization on health (see http://www.hado.net/index2.html). Emoto (2005, 1999) researched the effects positive and negative thoughts/images/verbalization had on the crystal structure of water. Positive communication resulted in formation of beautiful crystals in the water samples taken from around the world. Negative communication deformed crystal formation. If the body is made primarily from water, communication with ourselves has potential to affect the structure and function of the body. Changing images we hold in our mind's eye regarding cause and effect of pain is likely to decrease or eliminate pain.

Lance Armstrong visualized tumors leaving his body with the pain of voiding and vomiting induced by chemotherapy (Armstrong & Jenkins, 2001).

This visualization was likely extremely beneficial in ridding his body of cancer. Pain or its origins may be engulfed by white sharks, love, bugs, Pac-man–like creatures, highly pressurized fire hoses—anything the person can envision engulfing, eating, or in some way overcoming the pain. Clients may have destructive visions of removal of the pain, or visions that positively enhance healing mechanisms to take over abnormalities.

Appendices C–F contain scripts using guided imagery that are useful to relieve pain and anxiety.

Energy Therapies

Energy therapies are based on the premise that an imbalance in the energy field results in disruption of health (Krieger, 1979; Leonard, 1997; Oschman & Oschman, 1999; Slater, 2002). Rebalancing and smoothing the field with intention for the highest good of the individual removes or relieves pain. Examples of energy therapies include healing touch, Reiki, therapeutic touch, Shen, and polarity therapy, among others. Intention is the primary mechanism of action (Mentgen, 2001). Many energy therapies include specific hand movement protocols facilitating movement of the energy and the intention of connection to the universal field (Slater, 2002).

Disturbed energy field is a nursing diagnosis initiated with the North American Nursing Diagnosis Association (Ralph, Craft-Rosenberg, Herdman, & Lavin, 2005). The diagnosis is defined as disruption of the flow of energy surrounding a person's being, which results in a disharmony of the body, mind, and/or spirit. Characteristics defining the diagnosis are movement (wave/spike/tingling/dense/flowing), sounds (tones/words), temperature changes (warmth/coolness), visual changes (images/colors), and disruption of the field (vacant/hold/spike/bulge). Recognition of disrupted energy by internationally focused North American Nursing Diagnosis Association (NANDA) also lends credence to incorporation of the work in nursing and health care.

Energy therapies are conducted with the client fully clothed except for shoes. The client sits in a chair or lies on a padded table. Lights are dimmed, quiet music often accompanies, and the client relaxes during the treatment. Practitioners guide the treatment to allow the client to connect with the universal energy to facilitate their own healing.

The practitioner comes to the treatment centered—with a quiet body-mind-spirit, to attune fully to the needs of the client. Centering may be attained with breath work, imagery, meditation, and/or prayer to find an inner sense of equilibrium and stillness. Next the practitioner assesses the energy field of the person. Hands are held very lightly on or slightly above the surface of the body. The hands assess from the head to the feet. Sensory cues such as warmth, coolness, static, blockage, pulling, or tingling may be felt, along with visual, auditory, and intuitive cues. The practitioner notes the location and intensity of the cues, moving next to the intervention phase to treat them. Symmetrical flow of the practitioner's hands through the energy field of the client with intent for the person's highest good patterns or moves the energy for efficient use by the client. Energy may be transferred to areas of deficit or mobilized or repatterned from areas of congestion. The practitioner moves among these steps until the client's field is smooth and balanced or accomplishes as much as possible during the time frame available. Clients are grounded to the earth when the treatment is finished and the practitioner releases from their field.

Treatments last from 15 to 60 minutes typically, with a brief rest period after. The client and practitioner discuss what was experienced and found in the energy field after the treatment. Clients are often taught self-care techniques to practice on their own between scheduled appointments.

Energy therapies are integrated with traditional therapies or used as a standalone treatment. Practitioners use their hands with light or near-body touch to help clear, balance, and energize the human energy system, thus promoting healing for the mind, body, and/or spirit. Balanced energy correlates with decreased pain and anxiety, as will be discussed in the evidence base section. Healing touch and therapeutic touch are two specific energy therapies that will be discussed further.

Healing touch (HT) is an umbrella term for a program offering multiple energy modalities used for specific forms of disruption, of which pain is a primary focus. Healing touch is taught in five levels, and participants may attain certification upon completion of the levels and mentored practice (see http://www.healingtouchprogram.com/htp/faq.shtml). One of the modalities, the basic healing sequence, is very similar to therapeutic touch, being different primarily in the terms used describing the process of the techniques.

The therapeutic touch process (TT) was developed by Dr. Dolores Krieger, RN and Dora Kunz and introduced into nursing in the early 1970s. "Therapeutic Touch is a contemporary interpretation of several ancient healing practices, is an intentionally directed process of energy exchange during which the practitioner uses the hands as a focus for facilitating healing" (http://www.thera peutic-touch.org). Intention is again thought to be the primary mechanism of action. The practitioner facilitates the person to repattern their own energy toward health. Pain and anxiety decrease, relaxation is promoted, and the body's natural restorative processes are facilitated. In addition, TT can be used alone or with other healing modalities.

Evidence of Efficacy for Pain Relief—Healing Touch

At the current time, a wealth of studies on HT has been conducted (see http://www.healingtouch.net). However, very few studies are published and accessible for review. Many are listed on the Healing Touch International research database and have been reported at national conferences. Studies vary in sample size and are not focused primarily on elders, but do include subjects who are elderly. As noted earlier, studies do not fit the typical model in which every subject receives the exact same treatment; to do so may invoke harm. Instead, studies are conducted using a specific technique for a form of pain, and the outcome achieved is examined.

Experiments done on the effects HT has on clients yielded positive results A medical school elective using touch therapies fostered compassion in caregiving (Kemper, Larrimore, Dozier, & Woods, 2006). Umbreit (2000) and Wilkinson and colleagues (2002) found positive results with varying aspects of care-related problems in acute care settings. Measurable differences were found between agitation levels of clients with dementia who received HT compared with those who did not (Wang & Hermann, 2006). Clients experiencing painful cancer symptoms found therapeutic massage and HT to induce a relaxed state. These were more effective than presence alone or standard care in inducing physical relaxation, reducing pain, and improving mood states and fatigue (Post-White, Kinney, Savik, Bernsten, Wilcox, et al., 2003).

Healing touch was used after each radiation treatment in 25 women with breast cancer. The HT group demonstrated higher scores on all SF-36 subscales, with statistically significant higher scores than the control group for decrease of pain, vitality, and physical functioning (Cook, Guerrerio, & Slater, 2004).

Wardell and Weymouth (2004) reviewed studies conducted on HT. Nine studies covering chronic pain, orthopedic pain, and other pain syndromes were reviewed. The outcomes of the studies indicate healing touch is effective for pain management in many situations. Seven studies indicated decreased pain, one no change, and one showed decreased pain when healing touch was paired with reflexology.

A study of clients receiving hospice care showed that healing touch experienced "amelioration of physical symptoms," while those who received standard hospice care declined physically (Ziembroski, Gilbert, Bossarte, & Guldberg, 2003, p. 150). Clients who received healing touch in addition to hospice care experienced slower decline in physical functioning and had an easier time with interpersonal relationships than those who received standard hospice care (Ziembroski, Gilbert, Bossarte, & Guldberg, 2003).

Wardell (2000) conducted a qualitative study on the specific HT technique called trauma release. The trauma release technique fostered complete remission of pain for some of the subjects—both physically and psychologically—and improved pain for most others. The study "supports the belief that energy work is a self-healing process" (p. 27) that assists the person to repattern their response to situations and stimuli. Some participants experienced continued further recovery across time after treatments ended.

Healing touch case studies were analyzed across varying medical diagnoses (Scandrett-Hibden, Hardy, & Mentgen, 1999). In each case, clients with a specific medical diagnosis/problem had five to six treatments each. The authors highlight the energetic assessments/findings and treatments of the problems. Common energy imbalances were identified within groups. For example, people with breast cancer had a block in the second chakra. Chakras are energy centers of the body and its surrounding energy field, points where the flow of energy moves through the body and its field. A connection between these centers, the endocrine glands underlying them, and emotional regulation has been theorized (Gerber, 2000). The second chakra is located halfway between the pubic bone and the umbilicus and is theorized to relate to how we deal with others personally, in working and sexual relationships (Gerber, 2000).

Healing touch treatments (from Scandrett-Hibden et al., 1999, case studies) were given based on the practitioner's insight into the energetic assessment and according to established protocol for practice of HT. The authors reviewed how the energy fields became more balanced and symmetrical with each treatment and summarized changes clients experienced. Some clients experienced no change or died if they were terminally ill. However, the majority of cases showed positive outcomes. Terminally ill clients, who went on to die, expressed that they could feel healing and peace as they transitioned to death. This work is foundational to further research on the type of treatments needed in specific situations and the number and frequency of treatments needed to relieve pain, promote healing, and foster well-being in clients.

Evidence of Efficacy for Pain Relief—Therapeutic Touch

Much of the energy research published to date has been done on therapeutic touch. Research involving TT for pain relief is extensive. Some studies provide evidence on areas that are affected by pain, such as sleep, quality of life, and functional ability.

Pain relief was researched directly in nine studies (Denison, 2004; Gordon, Merenstein, D'Amico, & Hudgens, 1998; Peck, 1997; Biley, 1996; Keller & Bzdek,

1986; Meehan, 1993; Silva, 1996; Turner, Clark, Gauthier, & Williams, 1998; Spross, 1999). Each study showed decreased pain with the use of TT. Subjects in the studies had pain from varying causes—arthritis, fibromyalgia, phantom pain, headache, complex abdominal surgery, and burns.

Anxiety was reduced using TT in 22 studies. Anxiety is a key component of the pain-anxiety-tension cycle (Ferrell-Torey & Glick, 1993; Gagne & Toye, 1994; Heidt, 1981; Quinn, 1984; Simington & Laing, 1993; Giasson & Bouchard, 1998; Guerrero, 1985; Heidt, 1981; LaFreniere, Mutus, Cameron, Tannous, Giannotti, et al., 1999; Leb, 1997; Lin & Taylor, 1998; Newshan & Schuller-Civitella, 2003; Olson, Sneed, Bonadonna, Ratliff, & Dias, 1992; Quinn, 1984; Samarel, 1992; Simington & Laing, 1993; Wilkinson, 1999; Samarel, 1992; Samarel, Fawcett, Davis, & Ryan, 1998; Snyder, Egan, & Burns, 1995; Woods, Craven, & Whitney, 1996; Wright, 1995; Verret, 2001). Reducing or eliminating anxiety affects pain management. The study by Parkes was alone in not improving anxiety. Parkes's study tried to control a normal emotional reaction to a stressor and it is suspected that is the reason why it was not effective. In addition to relieving anxiety, studies found increased well-being, improved sleep, comfort, calmness, and enhanced well-being serendipitously. All of these contribute to pain reduction.

Wound healing was studied by four authors, and in one analytic review (Daley, 1997; Wirth, 1992; Wirth, Barrett, & Eidelman, 1994; Wirth, Richardson, Martinez, Eidelman, & Lopez 1996). Studies by Wirth provide randomized double-blind evidence of wound-healing properties of TT. One study by Wirth did not show improvement; multiple therapies were in use and may have confounded results. Wound healing often contributes to reduction of pain.

Functional ability improved in two very similar studies (Gordon et al., 1998; Peck, 1998). Arthritis patients found that the decrease of pain after TT improved their functional ability.

Some studies have looked specifically at an outcome, only to find that there were other things that occurred in a beneficial manner in addition to the outcome that was being researched. The most common examples of these "serendipitous" findings are emotional well-being, quality of life, and sleep improvement. These quality-of-life factors are substantially affected in persons with pain. Improved well-being and quality of life was reported in two studies (Giasson & Bouchard, 1998; Peck, 1997, 1998). Heidt (1991) and Peck (1998) reported improvement in sleep with the use of TT. Therapeutic touch can be a significant factor creating improvement in pain and subsequently quality of life.

Resource Base for Training and Credentialing in Therapies

The American Holistic Nurses' Certification Corporation (AHNCC) began certifying nurses in holistic nursing in 1997. There are two board certification examinations—the basic HN-BC exam and the advanced level AHN-BC. The American Holistic Nurses Association (AHNA) announced in November 2006 that its holistic nursing specialty of practice certification was recognized through the American Nurse Association (http://ahna.org/new/specialty.html). Supporting this new specialty focus, the ANA provides a leading edge for nursing to transform health care and provide help to clients where it has been lacking in the past. The American Board of Holistic Medicine has certified medical doctors and doctors of osteopathy in holism since 1996 (http://www.holisticboard.org/aboutus.html).

Health care providers can become familiar with complementary therapy practitioners in their community, learning their credentials and experiencing for themselves the quality of the practitioners' work. Appropriate credentialing is the basis by which the public can be assured that the provider has knowledge and mentored clinical practice experience for their work. Providers of complementary therapies may offer other services for which there is no certification or for which they do not hold certification. Nurses should encourage clients to interview the provider before receiving care to determine if the provider carries credentials for the work they do, and to get to know them. It is up to the client to determine whether or not the therapy is appropriate by learning about the therapy from literature and Web sites. Talking with the provider before receiving treatment will assist the client to determine whether or not to try the treatment.

Health care providers need knowledge of the evidence base to direct client questions. However, caution is needed—reading two or three studies about any therapy (medically based or complementary) does not verify or validate efficacy. Read studies, experience the therapies, and ask practitioners to teach about the literature and evidence base for their therapy.

Health care providers should make respectful inquiry of their clients regarding what complementary therapies are in use. Doing so facilitates respect for client decision-making and praises initiative in managing their own personal care. Clients should also let the complementary provider know that they are seeking help from a medical practitioner. Other than conducting research studies, the best way to determine which therapy is making a difference in our health is to look at the whole, complementary therapies and medical therapies, used in an integrated fashion. If the medical provider is only aware of the medical therapies being used, they may inaccurately determine a "success or failure" to be from the medical therapy. The same "success or failure" can be attributed to a complementary therapy if the complementary provider is unaware that the client is simultaneously seeking care from a medical provider. If one takes a holistic approach, this communication is seamless for all parties involved.

In addition, medical providers and complementary providers can help the client be aware of side effects and interactions that result from the integration of medical and complementary therapies. That is not to say that complementary therapies should not be used with medical therapies; quite the contrary. It is often easy enough to monitor specific health care outcomes while complementary and medical therapies are integrated. But for integration of complementary and medical therapies to be successful, the client, complementary provider, and the medical provider have to talk together.

Credentials can be found on Web sites for national organizations supporting specific therapies. Credentials for select therapies covered in this chapter can be found in Table 8.2. Contact the organizations to learn where to obtain training in the therapies.

SUMMARY

Evidence supports the efficacy of mind-body and energy therapies for pain relief and shows that clients are using them widely, regardless of medical reference for complementary therapies. Adaptation of the WHO pain ladder to include complementary therapies at every level would facilitate improved management of pain for most clients. Implementation of complementary therapies will increase pain control for clients and decrease anxiety. Breaking the pain-tension-anxiety cycle improves physical functioning and socialization, providing clients with an increased ability to remain active in their roles in life, and contribute to their communities.

Health care providers must learn about the complementary therapies the public is using—the evidence base, the experience of the treatments, and the practice of complementary therapies. Knowledge portrayed in discussions with clients improves credibility of the health care providers and increases trust in clients. Assisting clients to navigate complementary modalities improves health care and gives health care providers a realistic view of what really is working. Interested nurses, doctors, and other providers can attain certification as holistic providers, increasing their ability to look at the whole client and their needs. Health care is changing—health care providers can lead the way.

TABLE 8.2   Credentials for Selected Therapies

Therapy	Credential	Certification Body
Healing touch	CHTP or CHTI	Healing Touch, International HEALING TOUCH PROGRAM™ PO Box 16189 Golden, Colorado 80402 Phone: 303-989-0581 Fax: 303-985-9702 E-Mail: info@HealingTouchProgram.com Web site: http://www.healingtouchprogram.com/
Hypnotherapy	CHt	National Guild of Hypnotists, Inc. PO Box 308 Merrimack, NH 03054 Phone: 603-424-9438 E-mail: ngh@ngh.net Web site: http://www.ngh.net/
Massage	LMT or CMT	National Certification Board for Therapeutic Massage and Bodywork 1901 S. Meyers Rd., Suite 240 Oakbrook Terrace, IL 60181-5243 1-800-296-0664 Email: info@ncbtmb.com http://www.ncbtmb.com/
Therapeutic Touch	Qualified Therapeutic Touch Practitioner	NH-PAI, Inc. PO Box 158 Warnerville, NY 12187-0158 518-325-1185 877-32NHPAI nhpai@therapeutic-touch.org http://www.therapeutic-touch.org/
Holistic Nurse	HNC	American Holistic Nurses' Certification Corporation 811 Linden Loop Cedar Park, TX 78613 (877) 284-0998 AHNCC@flash.net. http://www.ahna.org/edu/certification.html
Holistic Doctor (MD or DO)		American Holistic Medical Association PO Box 2016 Edmonds, WA 98020 Phone: 425.967.0737 Fax: 425.771.9588 info@holisticmedicine.org http://www.holisticmedicine.org/

REFERENCES

Achterberg, J. (1985). *Imagery in healing: Shamanism and modern medicine.* Boston: Shambala.

Achterberg, J., Dossey, B., & Kolkmeier, L. (1994). *Rituals of healing: Using imagery for health and wellness.* New York: Bantam Books.

Administration on Aging. (2006). *The Administration on Aging gateway to the Older Americans Act Amendments of 2006.* Retrieved November 25, 2006, from http://www.aoa.gov/OAA2006/Main_Site/index.aspx.

Armstrong, L., & Jenkins, S. (2001). *It's not about the bike, my journey back to life.* New York: Berkeley Publishing.

Astin, J. (2004). Mind-body therapies for the management of pain. *Clinical Journal of Pain, 20*(1), 27–32.

Biley, F. (1996). Rogerian science, phantoms, and therapeutic touch: Exploring potentials. *Nursing Science Quarterly, 9*(4), 165–169.

Bodane, C., & Brownson, K. (2002). The growing acceptance of complementary and alternative medicine. *Health Care Manager, 20*(3), 11–21.

Borneman, T., & Browne-Salzman, K. (2006). Meaning in illness. In B. Ferrell (Ed.) *Textbook of palliative nursing.* Oxford, NY: Oxford University Press.

Cook, C., Guerrerio, J., & Slater, V. (2004). Healing touch and quality of life in women receiving radiation treatment for cancer: a randomized controlled trial. *Alternative Therapies, 10*(3), 34–41.

Daley, B. (1997). Therapeutic touch, nursing practice and contemporary cutaneous wound healing research. *Journal of Advance Nursing, 25*(6), 1123–1132.

Denison, B. (2004, May–June). "Touch the pain away": New research on therapeutic touch and person with fibromyalgia syndrome. *Holistic Nursing Practice, 18,* 142–151.

Edgar, I. (1999). The imagework method in health and social science research. *Qualitative Health Research, 9*(2), 198–212.

Eisenberg, D., Davis, R., Ettner, S., Appel, S., Wilkey, S., Van Rompay, M., et al. (1998). Trends in alternative medicine use in the United States, 1990–1997: Results of a follow-up national survey. *Journal of the American Medical Association, 280,* 1569–1575.

Emoto, M. (1999). *Messages from water.* Netherlands: Hado Publishing.

Emoto, M. (2005). *The true power of water: Healing and discovering ourselves.* Hillsboro, OR: Beyond Words Publishing.

Ferrell-Torey, A., & Glick, O. (1993). The use of therapeutic massage as a nursing intervention to modify anxiety and the perception of cancer pain. *Cancer Nursing, 16*(2), 93–101.

Freeman, L. (2004). *Mosby's complementary and alternative medicine: A research based approach.* Philadelphia: Mosby.

Gagne, D., & Toye, R. (1994). The effects of therapeutic touch and relaxation in reducing anxiety. *Archives of Psychiatric Nursing, 8*(3), 184–189.

Gerber, R. (2000). *Vibrational medicine for the 21st century.* New York: Eagle Brook, Harper/Collins.

Giasson, M., & Bouchard, L. (1998). Effect of therapeutic touch on the well being of persons with terminal cancer. *Journal of Holistic Nursing, 16*(3), 383–398.

Gordon, A., Merenstein, J., D'Amico, F., & Hudgens, D. (1998). The effects of therapeutic touch on subjects with osteoarthritis of the knee. *The Journal of Family Practice, 47*(4), 271–277.

Guerrero, M. A. (1985). The effects of therapeutic touch on state-trait anxiety level of oncology subjects. *Masters Abstracts, 24,* AAD13–23756.

Heidt, P. (1981). Effect of Therapeutic Touch on anxiety level of hospitalized subjects. *Nursing Research, 30*(1), 32–37.

Heidt, P. (1991). Helping subjects to rest: Clinical studies in therapeutic touch. *Holistic Nurse Practice, 5*(4), 57–66.

Huddleston, P. (1996). *Prepare for surgery, heal faster: A guide of mind-body techniques.* Cambridge, MA: Angel River Press.

Kazanowski, M., & Laccetti, M. (2002). *Pain.* Thorofare, NJ: SLACK, Inc.

Keller, E., & Bzdek, V. (1986). Effects of therapeutic touch on tension headache pain. *Nursing Research, 35*(2), 101–106.

Kemper, K., Larrimore, D., Dozier, J., & Woods, C. (2006). Impact of a medical school elective cultivating compassion through touch therapies. *Complementary Health Practice Review, 11*(1), 47–56.

Krieger, D. (1979). *Therapeutic touch: How to use your hands to help or heal.* New York: Prentice Hall.

LaFreniere, K., Mutus, B., Cameron, S., Tannous, M., Giannotti, M., Abu-Zahra, H., et al. (1999). Effects of therapeutic touch on biochemical and mood indicators in women. *Journal of Alternative and Complementary Medicine, 5*(4), 367–370.

Leb, C. (1997). *The effects of healing touch on depression.* Paper presented at the national conference for the American Holistic Nurses' Association, Olympia, WA, June 1997.

Leonard, G. (1997). Living energy: Subtle fields, subtle healing. *Noetic Science Review, 43,* 8. Retrieved January 3, 2008, from http://www.noetic.org/publications/review/issue43/r43_Leonard.html.

Lin, Y., & Taylor, A. (1998). Effects of therapeutic touch in reducing pain and anxiety in an elderly population. *Integrative Medicine, 1*(4), 155–162.

Meehan, M. (1993).Therapeutic touch and postoperative pain: A Rogerian research study. *Nursing Science Quarterly, 6*(2), 69–77.

Mentgen, J. (2001). Healing touch. *Nursing Clinics of North America, 36*(1), 143–157.

Myss, C. (2006). Caroline Myss Homepage. Retrieved November 22, 2006, from http://www.myss.com/

Newshan, G., & Schuller-Civitella, D. (2003, July–August). Large clinical study shows value of therapeutic touch program. *Holistic Nursing Practice, 17*(4), 189–192.

Olson, M., Sneed, N., Bonadonna, R., Ratliff, J., & Dias, J. (1992). Therapeutic touch and post-hurricane Hugo stress. *Journal of Holistic Nursing, 10,* 120–136.

Oschman, J., & Oschman, N. (1999). How energy therapies influence tissue healing. *Healing Touch Newsletter, 9*(3), 6–7.

Peck, S. (1997). The effectiveness of therapeutic touch for decreasing pain in elders with degenerative arthritis. *Journal of Holistic Nursing, 15*(2), 176–198.

Peck, S. (1998). The effectiveness of therapeutic touch for improving functional ability in elders with degenerative arthritis. *Nursing Science Quarterly, 11*(3), 123–132.

Post-White, J., Kinney, M., Savik, K., Bernsten, J., Wilcox, C., & Lerner, I. (2003). Therapeutic massage and healing touch improve symptoms in cancer. *Integrative Cancer Therapies, 2*(4), 332–344.

Quinn, J. (1984). Therapeutic touch as energy exchange: Testing the theory. *Advances in Nursing Science, 6*(2), 42–49.

Ralph, S., Craft-Rosenberg, M., Herdman, T. H., & Lavin, M. A. (2005). *Nursing diagnoses: Definitions and classification 2005–2006*. Philadelphia: NANDA International.

Samarel, N. (1992).The experience of receiving therapeutic touch. *Journal of Advanced Nursing, 17*, 651–657.

Samarel, N., Fawcett, J., Davis, M., & Ryan, F. (1998). Effects of dialogue and therapeutic touch on preoperative and postoperative experiences of breast cancer surgery: An exploratory study. *Oncology Nursing Forum, 25*(8), 1369–1376.

Scandrett-Hibdon, S., Hardy, C., & Mentgen, J. (1999). *Energetic patterns: Healing touch case studies* (Vol. 1). Denver: Colorado Center for Healing Touch.

Silva, C. (1996). The effects of relaxation touch on the recovery level of post-anesthesia abdominal hysterectomy subjects (abstract). *Alternative Therapies, 2*(4), 94.

Simington, J., & Laing, G. (1993). Effects of therapeutic touch on anxiety in the institutionalized elderly. *Clinical Nursing Research, 2*(4), 438–450.

Slater, V. (2002). Toward an understanding of the scientific bases of healing touch. *Healing touch: A guidebook for practitioners* (2nd ed.). Albany, NY: Delmar.

Sloman, R. (1995). Relaxation and the relief of cancer pain. *Nursing Clinics of North America, 30*, 697–709.

Snyder, M., Egan, E., & Burns, K. (1995). Interventions to decrease agitation behaviors in persons with dementia. *Journal of Gerontological Nursing, 21*(7), 34–40.

Spross, J. (1999). Nondrug intervention for pain management: The magnetic pain drain. *Developments in Supportive Cancer Care, 3*(3), 90–92.

Stephens, R. (1999). Imagery: A strategic intervention to empower clients part I: Review of research literature. *Clinical Nurse Specialist, 7*(4), 170–174.

Turner, J., Clark, A., Gauthier, D., & Williams, M. (1998). The effect of therapeutic touch on pain and anxiety in burn subjects. *Journal of Advanced Nursing, 28*(1), 10–20.

Tusek, D., Church, J., Strong, S., Grass, J., Fazio, V. (1997). A significant advance in the care of patients undergoing elective colorectal surgery. *The Cleveland Clinic Foundation, 40*, 172–178.

Umbreit, A. (2000). Healing touch: Applications in the acute care setting. *American Association of Critical-Care Nurses, 11*(1), 105–119.

Verret, P. (2001). *Healing touch and children with cerebral palsy.* Unpublished document.

Wang, K., & Hermann, C. (2006). Pilot study to test the effectiveness of healing touch on agitation in people with dementia. *Geriatric Nursing, 27*(1), 34–40.

Wardell, D. (2000). The trauma release technique. *Alternative and Complementary Therapies, 6*(1), 20–27.

Wardell, D., & Weymouth K. (2004). Review of studies of healing touch. *Journal of Nursing Scholarship, 36*(2), 147–154.

Wilkinson, D. (1999). *Clinical effectiveness of healing touch.* Unpublished manuscript.

Wilkinson, D., Knox, P., Chatman, J., Johnson, T., Barbour, N., Myles, Y., et al. (2002). The clinical effectiveness of healing touch. *The Journal of Alternative and Complementary Medicine, 8*(1), 33–47.

Wirth, D. (1992). The effect of non-contact therapeutic touch on the healing rate of full thickness dermal wounds. *Cooperative Connection, 13*(3), 2–8.

Wirth, D., Barrett, M., & Eidelman, W. (1994). Non-contact therapeutic touch and wound re-epithelialization: An extension of previous research. *Complementary Therapies in Medicine, 2*, 187–192.

Wirth, D., Richardson, J., Martinez, R., Eidelman, W., & Lopez, M. (1996). Non-contact therapeutic touch intervention and full-thickness cutaneous wounds: A replication. *Complementary Therapies in Medicine, 4*, 237–240.

Woods, D., Craven, R., & Whitney, J. (1996). The effect of therapeutic touch on disruptive behaviors of individuals with dementia of the Alzheimer type (abstract). *Alternative Therapies, 2*(4), 95–96.

World Health Organization. (2006). *Highlights.* Retrieved November 25, 2006, from http://www.who.int/en/

Wright, S. (1995). The use of therapeutic touch in the management of pain. *Nursing Clinics of North America, 22*(3), 705–714.

Zahourek, R. (1988). *Relaxation and imagery: Tools for therapeutic communication and intervention.* Philadelphia: Saunders Publishing.

Ziembroski, J., Gilbert, N., Bossarte, R., & Guldberg, M. (2003). Healing touch and hospice care. *Alternative and Complementary Therapies, 9*, 146–151.

APPENDIX A

Relaxation Script

Breathing Technique for Relaxation

Lie down with knees bent and spine straight, or sit in a chair. Uncross your arms and legs. Inhale slowly and deeply, feeling your abdomen slightly rise with each inhalation. Take some time to get in touch with your breath. Then, inhale through your nose, gently as though sniffing a delicate flower. Exhale gently through your mouth, making a gentle whooshing sound, while letting the air flow out as if you were gently blowing on a candle flame just enough to make it flicker. Continue breathing this way for 5–10 minutes, focusing on the sound of your breathing, the gentle rising and falling of your abdomen, and the sense of relaxation. Let thoughts or distractions pass in and out of your mind.

Practice at least 3–4 times a day. The more you practice the better you will become at relaxation.

Adapted with permission from Elsevier from Zahourek (1988).

APPENDIX B

Progressive Muscle Relaxation

Progressive muscle relaxation (PMR) was developed by Edmund Jacobson in the 1920s. It is widely used across health care to reduce pain and anxiety. Sit in a comfortable chair—reclining armchairs are ideal. Bed is okay too. Get as comfortable as possible—no tight clothes, no shoes, don't cross your legs. Take a deep breath; let it out slowly. Again. What you will be doing is alternately tensing and relaxing specific groups of muscles. After tension, a muscle will be more relaxed than prior to the tensing. Concentrate on the feel of the muscles, specifically the contrast between tension and relaxation. In time, you will recognize tension in any specific muscle and be able to reduce that tension. Don't tense muscles other than the specific group at each step. Don't hold your breath, grit your teeth, or squint! Breath slowly and evenly and think only about the tension-relaxation contrast. Each tensing is for 10 seconds; each relaxing is for 10 or 15 seconds. Count "1,000, 2,000 . . . " until you have a feel for the time span. Note that each step is really two steps—one cycle of tension-relaxation for each set of opposing muscles. Do the entire sequence once a day if you can, until you feel you are able to control your muscle tensions. Be careful: If you have problems with pulled muscles, broken bones, or any medical contraindication for physical activities, consult your doctor first.

1.   **Hands.** The fists are tensed; relaxed. The fingers are extended; relaxed.
2.   **Biceps and triceps.** The biceps are tensed (make a muscle—but shake your hands to make sure you are not tensing them into a fist); relaxed (drop your arm to the chair—really drop them). The triceps are tensed (try to bend your arms the wrong way); relaxed (drop them).

3. **Shoulders.** Pull them back (careful with this one); relax them. Push the shoulders forward (hunch); relax.

4. **Neck (lateral).** With the shoulders straight and relaxed, the head is turned slowly to the right, as far as you can; relax. Turn to the left; relax.

5. **Neck (forward).** Dig your chin into your chest; relax (bringing the head back is not recommended—you could break your neck).

6. **Mouth.** The mouth is opened as far as possible; relaxed. The lips are brought together or pursed as tightly as possible; relaxed.

7. **Tongue (extended and retracted).** With mouth open, extend the tongue as far as possible; relax (let it sit in the bottom of your mouth). Bring it back in your throat as far as possible; relax.

8. **Tongue (roof and floor).** Dig your tongue into the roof of your mouth; relax. Dig it into the bottom of your mouth; relax.

9. **Eyes.** Open them as wide as possible (furrow your brow); relax. Close your eyes tightly (squint); relax. Make sure you completely relax the eyes, forehead, and nose after each of the tensings—this is actually a toughy.

10. **Breathing.** Take as deep a breath as possible—and then take a little more; let it out and breathe normally for 15 seconds. Let all the breath in your lungs out—and then a little more; inhale and breathe normally for 15 seconds.

11. **Back.** With shoulders resting on the back of the chair, push your body forward so that your back is arched; relax. Be very careful with this one, or don't do it at all.

12. **Butt.** Tense the butt tightly and raise pelvis slightly off chair; relax. Dig buttocks into chair; relax.

13. **Thighs.** Extend legs and raise them about 6 inches off the floor or the foot rest—but don't tense the stomach; relax. Dig your feet (heels) into the floor or foot rest; relax.

14. **Stomach.** Pull in the stomach as far as possible; relax completely. Push out the stomach or tense it as if you were preparing for a punch in the gut; relax.

15. **Calves and feet.** Point the toes (without raising the legs); relax. Point the feet up as far as possible (beware of cramps—if you get them or feel them coming on, shake them loose); relax.

16. **Toes.** With legs relaxed, dig your toes into the floor; relax. Bend the toes up as far as possible; relax. Remain relaxed for a while. These exercises will not eliminate tension, but when it arises, if you have practiced, you will be able to tense-relax it away.

APPENDIX C

Guided Imagery Script #1 for General Pain Relief

General Pain Relief

As your mind becomes clearer and clearer, [insert your name]....Feel it becoming more and more alert. Somewhere deep inside of you, a brilliant light begins to glow. Sense this happening....The light grows brighter and more intense....This is the bodymind communication center. Breathe into it....Energize it with your breath. The light is powerful and penetrating, and a beam begins to grow from it. The beam shines into your body now as you prepare to reduce your perception of pain or discomfort.

As you allow your body to sink down into the surface on which you are resting....You might let your imagination travel directly to the area that has been causing you pain or discomfort....In your mind's eye see the blood vessels that bring healing oxygen, proteins, and other substances....See the blood vessels wrapping around and traveling through the area of pain, dropping off their healing compounds and absorbing all the waste products....If you have taken medication, notice how it appears within the blood vessels and within the area of injury....Many medications form crystals when they are dissolved in fluid. Can you imagine the medication as tiny jewel-like crystals?

As you continue to focus on the area of pain, is it possible to experience your own endorphins moving into the tissues?....You might imagine the endorphins like fluffy cotton, wrapping around the ends of the nerves, muffling and softening and even blocking out any pain messages....

If you feel that cold would help block your pain....Imagine breathing in an icy blue-green mist with each breath....Recall the color of icebergs or deep, frozen glaciers....Each time you breathe in....that mist wraps itself around and through the painful part, cooling the inflammation and decreasing the pain..... Feel the pain changing as you work with your imagery....You might also imagine bathing the painful area in a cool mountain stream....Notice how clear the cold water is....You can even see the colors and shapes of the tiny rocks deep in the icy stream....

If warmth seems to be best for your pain at this time, imagine stretching your body out on a soft warm blanket in a special, safe place outdoors....Listen to the sounds around you: birds calling to each other, the sound of water flowing nearby....Notice the wonderful fragrances of flowers and trees in bloom, perhaps the smell of freshly baked bread coming to you on a soft breeze....As you lie on the blanket, feeling secure and protected, feel the warmth of the sun soaking into your body....You might be able to imagine a smaller image of the sun deep within the area that has been causing you pain.....It might appear like a child's drawing of a smiling face within a golden circle....Or it may simply glow like a clear golden marble....Can you feel the rays of sunshine moving out into the surrounding tissue, warming and softening any tightness or discomfort?....Your small inner sun is there for you anytime you need to use it to soothe away pain or darkness....

Reprinted with permission from Achterberg et al. (1994).

APPENDIX D

Guided Imagery Script #2 Pain as an Object

Pain as an Object

Take some time now to simply be with your pain or discomfort.... Remember that your pain may be physical sensations or perhaps worries or fears.... Gather all of your pain into one particular spot, and begin to describe the pain silently.... Allow that pain to turn into an object.... Just see what comes to mind, as there is no right or wrong way to do this.... As you examine the object that has appeared, notice its size.... How wide is it from side to side?.... What is its depth from front to back?.... How tall is it from top to bottom.... Inches, feet, or more?.... Notice the texture of the object, and its color.... Does it make any vibration or sound?.... Do you think it is warm, hot, cool, or cold?.... Now begin to clearly identify the location of the pain in your body. Is it right on the surface of your skin, just below the surface, or perhaps very deep in your body?.... Identify exactly where it is....

Keeping your eyes gently closed, cup your hands together, palms up as if you were holding something in them.... Allow yourself mentally to place the pain object directly in the palms of your hands so you can examine it even more closely.... Have another look at the size of the object, its width, height, and thickness.... Feel the texture, and listen and feel for any sound or vibration coming from it.... Notice the color and temperature.... Now that you can hold the object, is it heavy or light?.... does it feel warm or cool to your hands?.... You may want to turn the object over in your hands to get more information about it....

If you can, take your hands and move them toward your body, as if you were placing the object back into your body.... If it is too painful to put back in your body, you may take some time to change any of its characteristics.... You may choose to throw part or all of it away, or make some changes that will allow you to live more comfortably with it.... You may wish to smooth out its surface or change its color.... Make any change you like and then return the object to its place within your body.

Reprinted with permission from Achterberg et al. (1994).

APPENDIX E

Guided Imagery Script #3 Ball of Pain

Ball of Pain

Give yourself some time to relax and let go of your tension.... Scan your body now for any aches, pains, tightness, or discomforts, both physical and emotional.... Now begin to gather up the pain into a ball.... A glowing, colored ball.... When you have the ball firmly in your mind's eye, begin to change the size of the ball, noticing how the shadings and intensity of the color change as you make the ball larger.... and then smaller.... Change the size of the ball several times, allowing it to become very large, larger than your entire body.... and then watch and feel it shrink down to a tiny dot of color.... Play with the possibilities of size, intensity, and color.... Move the ball of pain up to the surface of your skin now, and as you do so let some or all of the ball move through your skin and feel it resting gently on the surface of your body.... notice the size and color again as you image the ball beginning to float above the surface of your skin, floating up and away.... Moving across the room, and even drifting through the window or wall.... Imagine the ball that is your pain.... drifting out through the roof of the building and over the tops of the trees and buildings and finally disappearing from your sight.... Returning now to the feelings within your bodymind, again scan your body and become aware of any changes that have occurred, knowing that each time you practice this or another imagery exercise, you will become more adept at changing your pain....

Take a few slow, reenergizing breaths, and as you come back to full awareness of the room, know that whatever is right for you at this point in time is unfolding just as it should, and that you have done your best, regardless of the outcome....

Reprinted with permission from Achterberg et al. (1994).

APPENDIX F

Guided Imagery Script: Using the Senses to Relieve Pain

"Using the Senses to Relieve Pain"
By Sue Peck

The client describes their favorite place as being in the woods near their home, alongside the creek. Their favorite season to be at this place is the fall when leaves are changing. This place is in the northern Midwest.

Begin with relaxation, focusing on the breath for 3–5 minutes. Suggest the client settle into their chair/bed as though they are sitting or lying on a mossy surface alongside the creek. With their breath, they smell the spicy tang of the forest and the scent of fall flowers nearby. Once their breathing has calmed, eyes softened or closed, and the relaxation response is initiated, walk the client through their six senses and what they can remember and feel in this favorite place. The client does not need to give verbal feedback while you walk them through the script, just imagine in their mind, "being" there.

In the script below, "...." refers to pauses. Pauses are 5–15 seconds in length, unless marked as longer.

In your mind's eye, I want you to "see" everything that is around you. Begin with the trees with their branches stretching over you, protecting you from the sun, creating a comfortable resting place in the shade.... Truly take in your surroundings—the blueness of the creek as it gurgles and sparkles past you, warming in the sun's sparkling rays.... The velvety soft green of the moss you're resting upon.... and feel its softness on your skin, caressing you, helping you relax even more.... Now turn your eyes above to the leaves of the trees in all their multi-colored beauty. Reds, yellows, oranges, greens and browns dance in the breeze, swaying gently.... giving an occasional glimpse of the blue sky beyond.... Dressing the earth—spots of brilliant vibrant color over the healthful brown of the earth.... The rocks—gray, brown, black, tan.... studded with diamonds—crystals, reflecting the sun.... Birds swoop and dive from branch to branch, down to the ground.... The blue sky is cloudless, except for a wisp here and there—an angel's wing perhaps....

As you continue to "see," turn your attention to what you hear.... The babble of the creek, turning softly over the rocks.... the breeze sighing softly through the branches.... the coos of the doves, the warble of the robin, the hum of the hummingbird.... an acorn or pine cone being accepted back to the earth.... Squirrels chatter and with speedy pantomime jerks rollick over the trunk of the pine. . . . you become at peace with the silence, the solitude....

Your mind's eye will continue to see and hear while you turn your attention to what you can smell.... The spicy scent of the earth you noticed as you settled in.... crisp clear fall air.... the pines nearby warming with the sun, evoking rich scent.... Perhaps an animal nearby drifts its scent to you with the breeze.... the alluring aroma of the decaying vegetation softening the ground around you while fragrancing the air you breathe....

The taste of your picnic lunch just consumed.... Embellished with the spicy aroma of the forest surrounding you.... Water in your cup clears as it floats downward in your throat, washing away any tension as it rinses the mouth and throat....

Your mind's eye continues to see, hear, smell and taste.... while you turn your attention to what you feel.... the feel of the sun's rays on your body.... like pure white, cleansing energy moving through you from head to toes.... You rinse your fingers in the cold, clear creek, noticing its warmth when you'd expect more coolness.... The softness and comfort of the green mossy bed.... Its coolness.... Comfort just right for you.... You feel the earth with your toes and feet, with your backside.... having slipped your shoes off, contented into the earth's consolation ....Its heart pulsing up through you.... The fall air is crisp, yet the sun's warmth holds solace. . . . Breezes waft gently through your hair and around your shoulders. . . . The security of "your place". . . . The peace and serenity your place brings—the right place for you. . . . Meeting every need you have. . . . Whenever you go there. . . .

Take a few moments. . . . enjoy. . . . remember. . . . all that's here. . . . all you feel. . . . the glorious reprieve. . . . in this place. . . . Reprieve/Relaxation is here for you whenever you desire. . . . Pause 2–5 minutes. . . .

And now. . . . take a slow deep breath. . . . And another. . . . One more. . . . move your hands and feet, and "gently bring yourself back to the room."

Give the client time to refocus fully. As you debrief, ask how the images formed, if they fit the words you used or if the words could be changed to better fit their experience. The client may need to drink water or walk around the room to become fully grounded. Insufficient grounding can affect decision-making when the client returns to their home, work, or activity. Being fully grounded assists the client to function without risk.

Instruct the client to practice 2–4 times per day using a written script such as this that you develop with them, or a tape of the script, using music in the background. The more the client practices the better the pain relief that is achieved. Increased practice when experiencing mild pain increases clients' ability to use the imagery successfully when pain is worse. Most clients find practice decreases the incidence and severity of the pain overall.

CHAPTER 9

Pharmacologic Treatment

Michaelene P. Jansen

The treatment of acute and chronic pain in the older adult will often include one or more medications to treat the pain condition(s). One in five older Americans takes analgesic medications three or more times a week (AGS, 2002). In determining the medication that would be most appropriate for the older individual, the provider should review all the nonpharmacotherapeutic treatment options before prescribing or recommending pain medication. Pain is best managed with multiple modalities rather than just relying on one modality such as medications. Some providers are wary of prescribing pain medications in older adults due to the risk of adverse effects. However, it has been shown that older adults can safely use pain-modulating drugs (Xiang, Siccardi, Janagap, & Vorsanger, 2007; AGS, 2002).

The responsibility for prescribing the most appropriate medications lies with the prescriber. The average 75-year-old takes 6.5 medications per day. Not all prescribed medications may be appropriate for an older adult. A list of inappropriate medications for older adults was first published by Mark Beers in 1991, revised in 1997, and updated in 2002 to assist providers in making appropriate medication choices (Fick, Cooper, Wade, Waller, Maclean, et al., 2003). However, studies have shown that prescribing practices for older adults by providers have not improved since 1997 (Goulding, 2004). Table 9.1 lists the medications from Beers's criteria related to pain management.

TABLE 9.1   2002 Beers Criteria: Pain-Related Medications

Drug	Concern
Propoxyphene (Darvon®)	No advantage over acetaminophen for analgesic effect
Meperidine (Demerol®)	May cause confusion and not effective oral analgesic
Ketorolac (Toradol®)	Asymptomatic adverse GI effects
Muscle Relaxants (methocarbanol, carisprodol, metazalone, cyclobenzaprine)	Anticholinergic side effects, sedation and weakness
Long-term use of non-steroidal anti-inflammatory agents	High risk for GI bleeding, renal failure, high blood pressure, and heart failure

This chapter will examine the various classifications of pain medications and their applicability to the older population. A review of pharmacokinetics in the elderly is an important step in determining the best medication for an older individual. Polypharmacology is a major issue in the elderly, and drug, herbal, and food interactions must be considered prior to prescribing any type of pain medication. Relief of pain can be enhanced by frequent visits for reassurance and validation (AGS, 2002). Frequent monitoring and review of over-the-counter (OTC) and herbal medications is crucial. Every effort should be made to keep pain management plans simple and costs manageable.

PHARMACOKINETICS

Pharmacokinetics related specifically to aging must be considered in any pain management plan. Drug distribution is altered in older adults due to changes in blood flow to organs, protein binding, and body composition (Gloth, 2001). Older adults have a loss of total body fluid and higher fat distribution compared to younger adults. Renal and hepatic function declines with aging. Renal clearance decreases approximately 1% per year between the ages of 50 and 100. The decline in the renal function can decrease the excretion of the drug and its metabolites, resulting in increased serum concentration of the drug. Blood flow to the liver decreases with age and affects drug metabolism. Since most drugs are metabolized by the liver, the net result is an increase in

TABLE 9.2   Factors Affecting Drug Dosages in Older Adults

Factor Related to Aging	Pharmacologic Effect
Decreased renal function	• Decreased renal excretion of drug and metabolite • Increased serum drug levels • Drug accumulation
Decreased hepatic function	• Decreased metabolism • Drug accumulation
Decreased albumin	• Higher levels of unbound drug • Toxicity
Altered target organ sensitivity	• Iatrogenic effects
Drug interactions	• Increased or decreased serum drug levels

drug accumulation. Therefore, caution must be used with any long-acting or extended release drugs.

In addition to decreased liver and renal function, older adults are more likely to have decreased protein levels, particularly albumin. Many drugs bind to protein. If the drugs cannot bind to proteins, more active unbound drug is available, resulting in increased drug effect or toxicity. Sensitivity of target organs may be altered in aging, allowing iatrogenic effects to occur. Use of multiple drugs, common in the elderly, causes many interactions, some undesirable. Although not a physiological effect, compliance may also play a role in pharmacotherapeutics in that the therapeutic goal may not be reached. Table 9.2 summarizes the factors that can affect drug dosages in older adults.

Several other aspects of aging may also play a role in managing pain with pharmacologic agents. Cortical and subcortical changes in the brain cause increased sensitivity to analgesics. In addition, pulmonary reserve is also diminished, allowing little margin for respiratory depression. Changes in the amygdala and frontal cortex that occur in some dementias influence the affective/motivational component of pain.

MANAGING PAIN WITH
PHARMACOTHERAPEUTIC AGENTS

A general principle associated with prescribing medications for the older adult is to "start low and go slow." The same is true for prescribing analgesics for the elderly. Analgesics can be safely administered to older adults if basic principles are followed. Basic principles for prescribing analgesics to older adults include:

- Have a definitive diagnosis to know where the pain generators are located.
- Begin with the least potent drug recommended for a particular pain condition.
- Review all medications, supplements, and herbal medications for possible interactions.
- Follow patient closely for frequent monitoring of pain relief, function, and side effects.
- Anticipate side effects and be proactive in preventing them.

The World Health Organization (WHO) developed a three-step analgesic ladder for treating cancer pain. It has also been adapted to treat nonmalignant pain. The analgesic ladder begins with nonopioid analgesics along with adjuvant and complementary therapies. Adjuvant therapies are drugs that have been developed for other primary purposes but have been found to alter, attenuate, or modulate pain perception (AGS, 2002). It is noted that these drugs may be considered adjuvant for cancer pain, but they are often the drug of choice for some neuropathic conditions.

If pain persists after trying medications in step one of the WHO analgesic ladder, the second step suggests that opioids for mild to moderate pain be tried. Nonopioid analgesics, and adjuvant and complementary therapies may also be continued. If pain relief is not achieved with therapies outlined in step two, then opioids for moderate to severe pain should be used. These medications are most beneficial if extended release formulations are used to maintain a therapeutic drug level. Previous classes of analgesics and nonpharmacologic therapies should also be used. Exhibit 9.1 illustrates the well-known WHO analgesic ladder.

Nonopioid Pain Medications

Nonopioid analgesics are indicated for mild to moderate pain. Typically, acetaminophen, nonsteroidal anti-inflammatory drugs, tramadol, and corticosteroids make up this group of analgesics. These medications are indicated for mild to moderate musculoskeletal pain, minor trauma, or postoperative pain.

Nonsteroidal Anti-Inflammatory Drugs (NSAIDs)

Nonsteroidal anti-inflammatory drugs (NSAIDs) inhibit the enzyme cyclooxygenase (COX), preventing the conversion of arachidonic acid to prostaglandin

EXHIBIT 9.1 WHO PAIN RELIEF LADDER

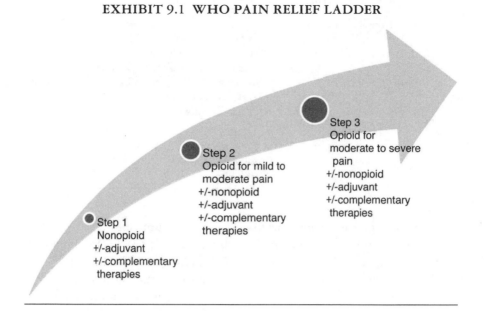

Step 3
Opioid for
moderate to severe
pain
+/-nonopioid
+/-adjuvant
+/-complementary
therapies

Step 2
Opioid for mild to
moderate pain
+/-nonopioid
+/-adjuvant
+/-complementary
therapies

Step 1
Nonopioid
+/-adjuvant
+/-complementary
therapies

or thromboxane A2 (Dahl, 2005). Prostaglandins and thromboxane A2 are chemical mediators released when cells are damaged or inflammation occurs. There are two isoforms of COX. COX-1 is responsible for maintaining the stability of the gastrointestinal (GI) lining and plays a role in platelet aggregation. COX-2 is induced in inflamed tissue.

There are two classes of NSAIDs, nonselective and selective COX-2 inhibitors. The nonselective NSAIDs inhibit COX-1 and COX-2. Medications in this class include aspirin, nonacetylated salicylates, and nonsalicylate NSAIDs. Table 9.3 provides examples of nonselective NSAIDs. The selective COX-2 inhibitor class currently has one medication available, celecoxib (Celebrex®). Two other drugs (refecoxib and valdecoxib) in this category have been recalled due to undesirable side effects.

All NSAIDS have analgesic, antipyretic, and anti-inflammatory properties. This class of medication works well for mild to moderate pain. However, there is an analgesic ceiling on NSAIDs. If one subclass fails to be effective another class may be beneficial. The choice of NSAID depends on cost, dosage, toxicity, side effects, and half-life. The selective COX-2 inhibitors are recommended for patients with high gastrointestinal risk. Prior authorization and failure on the nonselective NSAIDs needs to be established. Conflict occurs in prescribing NSAIDs for older adults because long-term use of nonselective NSAIDs is not recommended (Fick et al., 2003). However, many formularies will not

TABLE 9.3   Non-Selective NSAIDs Classes

Nonsalicylates	Profens (ibuprofen, ketoprofen)
	Indoles (indomethacin)
	Fenamates (diclofenac)
	Napththyalkanones (nabumetone)
	Indole acetic acids (ketorolac)
	Acetic acid derivatives (etodolac)
	Oxicams (piroxicam)
Salicyalates	Aspirin
	Choline magnesium trisalicylate
	Salsalate
	Diflunisal

grant prior approval for the selective COX-2 inhibitor until a nonselective NSAID is trialed for a certain length of time. Selective COX-2 inhibitors are often a higher-tiered drug with higher copay. Selective COX-2 inhibitors may also be contraindicated if the older person has cardiovascular disease.

There are several side effects associated with the use of non steroidal anti-inflammatory agents. COX-1 is responsible for the stability of the GI lining, so blocking this enzyme can result in gastrointestinal bleeding. Proton pump inhibitors help prevent GI bleeding with use of NSAIDs; however, it is often difficult to justify the use and cost of an additional medication to cover side effects of another drug. The selective COX-2 inhibitors have a lower occurrence of GI bleeding unless an individual also takes a low-dose daily aspirin, and then the incidence of ulcers is comparable (Strand, 2006).

Other side effects associated with NSAIDs use include effects on the central nervous system, heart, kidneys, liver, and platelets. There have been numerous studies and papers discussing the risk of cardiovascular disease and use of COX-2 NSAIDs. There have been varying results related to incidence of arrhythmias, heart failure, myocardial infarction, and stroke with use of COX-2 inhibitors (White, 2007). One Canadian study demonstrated increased incidence of acute myocardial infarction (MI) in patients with no history of MI (Levesque, Brophy, & Zhang, 2005) with the use of now recalled refecoxib (Vioxx®). Further analysis determined that the highest risk for MI in older adults occurred within one week of starting the medication (Levesque, Brophy, & Zhang, 2006).

Questions have also been raised regarding whether or not NSAIDs delay healing following surgery. Many surgeons limit use of NSAIDs following spinal fusion surgeries or orthopedic procedures, based on animal studies. However, there does not appear to be delayed healing in patients (Dahl, 2005).

Parenteral ketorolac, the only parenteral NSAID available, is a potent and effective analgesic postoperatively. The question of impaired wound and bone healing persists, however. Parenteral ketorolac has high GI toxicity and is indicated only for short-term use.

Topical NSAIDs are limited, and some preparations need to be compounded. Topical non-steroidal agents have shown similar results to oral medications in clinical trials and may be beneficial without the systemic effects.

Tramadol (Ultram®)

Tramadol is a unique medication in that it is a mu opioid agonist and a serotonin/norepinepherine reuptake inhibitor. Tramadol is not effective for acute pain and does not possess any anti-inflammatory effects. Caution must be used when administered with selective serotonin reuptake inhibitors due to risk of serotonin syndrome. Extended release tramadol dosed daily is now available and appears to be well tolerated (Gana, Pascual, Fleming, Schein, Janagap, et al., 2006)

Corticosteroids

Use of corticosteroids should be limited in older adults due to the potential adverse effects of the drugs. The primary indication for steroid use to control pain is in the treatment of rheumatoid arthritis. In addition to suppressing the hypothalamus-pituitary axis, corticosteroids can also cause hyperglycemia and depression.

Adjuvant Therapies

There are several categories of medications that are useful in treating pain, particularly neuropathic pain. Adjuvant medications are drugs that have primary applications other than as an analgesic. Examples of categories of adjuvant medications include antidepressants, anticonvulsants, N-methyl-D-aspartic acid (NMDA) receptor antagonists, and alpha 2 agonists. Muscle relaxants, hypnotics, and anxiolytics have been beneficial in the multimodality approach to treating pain.

Antidepressants

Although selective serotonin reuptake inhibitors prevent the reuptake of serotonin, a neurotransmitter involved in pain transmission, they have not shown benefit in treating pain. However, the dual reuptake inhibitors such as ven-laxafine (Effexor) and duloxetine (Cymbalta) have demonstrated effectiveness in treating neuropathic pain. The tricyclic antidepressants have been used for some time in treating neuropathic pain and fibromyalgia.

Tricyclic Antidepressants   Tricyclic antidepressants such as amitriptyline, imipa-ramine, climipramine, nortriptyline, desipramine, and maprotyiine have been used primarily in treating diabetic neuropathy and fibromyalgia. The tricyclic antidepressants are given in low, nonantidepressant doses, almost always in the evening prior to bedtime due to the sedating effect of the medications even in low doses. The tricyclic antidepressants have a narrow therapeutic index and are not tolerated very well by older adults due to the many side effects, including the anticholinergic effects.

Side effects include sedation, hypotension, dry mouth, blurred vision, uri-nary retention, constipation, atrial arrhythmias, and weight gain. Many older adults are taking antihypertensive agents, and the addition of a tricyclic anti-biotic increases their risk of falling.

Serotonin and Norepinephrine Reuptake Inhibitors   Two drugs fall within this classification, venlafaxine (Effexor®) and duloxetine (Cymbalta®). Of the two drugs, duloxetine is used more frequently. It is the first drug to be approved for both depression and neuropathic pain, specifically diabetic neuropathy.

The mechanism of action for duloxetine is not fully understood. Duloxetine has demonstrated a decrease in neuropathic pain associated with diabetic neu-ropathy. Duloxetine is contraindicated in chronic liver disease, alcohol abuse, and uncontrolled angle-closure glaucoma. Side effects include suicidality, hepatotoxicy, seizures, and mania. Duloxetine can be used in the elderly but caution is advised.

Anticonvulsants

Anticonvulsants have been widely used as an adjuvant medication for pain. Several anticonvulsants have been used in the treatment of migraine headache prophylaxis. Two drugs, gabapentin (Neurontin®) and pregabalin (Lyrica®) have been very useful in treating neuropathic pain. Although pregabalin has been used in Europe for over 10 years, it has only been released recently in the United States.

Gabapentin reduces the influx of calcium by blocking the channels. The decrease in calcium release decreases the amount of glutamate released from the nerve endings. Although gabapentin does not have a specific indication for neuropathic pain, it is widely used and monitored closely. This medication needs to be titrated slowly upward as well as downward. A typical starting dose for adults is 300 mg daily, then titrating every three days to 300 mg three times a day. A dose of 1,800 mg is usually needed to obtain relief. A long-acting formulation may allow higher doses. In the elderly population, the dose needs to begin with 100 mgs, typically at night, and increased by 100 mg every three days.

Side effects include sedation, dizziness and nausea, ataxia, fatigue, edema, and blurred image. Serious less common side effects include leukopenia, thrombosis, dyskinesa, and depression.

Pregabalin (Lyrica®) has analgesic, antianxiety, and anticonvulsant properties. It is approved for use in treating diabetic peripheral neuropathy, postherpetic neuralgia, fibromyalgia, and as an adjunct medication for partial seizures. Pregabalin has six times the binding capacity of gabapentin with rapid onset, and few drug interactions. Pregabalin needs to be used with caution if the patient is concurrently on a thiazolidinedione such as pioglitazone (Actos®) or rosiglitazone (Avandia®) due to edema. The risk of seizure activity increases if the drug is withdrawn rapidly. Other side effects include dizziness, somnolence, dry mouth, blurred vision, weight gain, and decreased concentration or attention. The maximum dose of pregabalin for diabetic neuropathy is 300 mg/day, whereas the maximum dose for post-herpetic neuralgia is 600 mg per day divided in 2 or 3 doses. The maximum dose for treating fibromyalgia is 450 mg per day.

Alpha 2 Agonists

Clonidine is an adrenergic agonist that can be helpful in some neuropathic pain conditions, particularly post-herpetic neuralgia and chronic regional pain syndrome. It is most helpful in situations where the pain is refractory to opioid medications. Clonidine is available in oral and transdermal forms. Clonidine has also been used in the withdrawal of opiate analgesics. It is important to monitor the older adult for hypotension, rebound hypertension, and dizziness. Clonidine would not be considered a first-line medication for an older adult due to these side effects.

Tizanidine (Zanaflex®) is another central-acting alpha 2 agonist. It is frequently thought of as a muscle relaxant. Tizanidine is used in the treatment of muscle spasms, spasticity, neuropathic pain, and there is some question as to whether or not it is effective in treating fibromyalgia. Tizanidine can be quite hepatotoxic, so it needs to be used with great caution in older adults. The analgesic dose for tizanidine ranges between 4 and 40 mg per day. A typical dose is usually 6–12 mg per day.

Antispasmotics

Baclofen is a gamma aminobutryic acid (GABA) beta receptor agonist. It binds to presynaptic receptors in the dorsal horn and brain stem, as well as cortical areas. It is used primarily to treat spasticity but is also used in treating neuropathic pain. Baclofen has been used more in recent years not only with spasticity related to spinal cord injuries, but also with neuromuscular diseases such as cerebral palsy, stroke, and traumatic brain injury. Baclofen can be given orally but also can be given intrathecally as a continuous infusion for severe spasticity. The main side effect is related to orthostasis, which puts the older adult at risk for falls. Baclofen needs to be tapered when discontinued, as seizures can occur with sudden withdrawal of the medication. Oral doses of baclofen range from 30–200 mg/day in divided doses.

Muscle Relaxants

The use of muscle relaxants is very controversial in terms of efficacy. There is no consistent data supporting their use. Muscle relaxants are indicated for short-term use for pain and muscle spasm. These medications are not indicated for spasticity. These drugs are central acting and cause somnolence, putting the older adult at risk for falling. Drugs in this category include methocarbamol (Robaxin®), carisoprodol (Soma®), chlorzoxazone (Parafon®), and metaxalone (Skelaxin®). These medications should be avoided in older adults.

Cyclobenzaprine (Flexeril®) is the most commonly known muscle relaxant. It is a central acting tricyclic medication. The drug is classified as an analgesic, not an antidepressant. However, cyclobenzeprine should not be used with other tricyclic agents. Somnolence is a major side effect of this drug, along with increased heart rate and anticholinergic effects. Typical dosing is 10 mg every eight hours and it needs to be used very cautiously in older adults.

Benzodiazepines

Benzodiazepines should be avoided in older adults and this drug category is on the updated Beers list for inappropriate medications for older adults. However, benzodiazepines, particularly short-acting benzodiazepines, are often found on medication lists of older adults. Benzodiazepines are often prescribed when a patient presents with coexisting anxiety. Benzodiazepines enhance the action of GABA, an inhibitory neurotransmitter in pain transmission. The two drugs that are seen most often on medication lists are lorazepam (Ativan®)

and clonazepam (Klonopin®). Clonazepam is given at night to facilitate sleep and also has an analgesic property. However, sedation and dizziness are common side effects, and physical dependence can occur with long-term use of these medications. These medications should not be taken with alcohol due to alcohol's effects on GABA receptors. Alprazolam (Xanax®) and diazepam (Valium®) should not be used in older adults.

Topical Analgesics

Topical analgesic creams such as lidocaine or capsaicin may be beneficial as an adjunctive therapy for certain pain syndromes such as peripheral diabetic neuropathy or post-herpetic neuralgia. Lidocaine cream (3%, 4%) or patches (5%) have been helpful for localized arthritic pain and post-herpetic neuralgia. One study comparing 5% lidocaine patches with celecoxib was cut short due to the efficacy of lidoderm (Gammaitoni, Oleka, & Gould, 2006). Capsaisin, derived from hot chili peppers, contains substance P, an inhibitory neurotransmitter involved in pain transmission and is available for topical application. A commercial product (Axsain®) combines 0.25% capsaicin cream in a lidocaine-containing vehicle. One caution with use of capsaicin products is that there is burning at the site of administration. If the person does not use gloves or an applicator, the person can experience burning on other parts of the body where it is touched, for example the eyes.

Ziconotide

Ziconotide (Prialt®) is a new development in treating refractory pain. The medication blocks the N-type calcium channels on nociceptive nerves in the spinal cord. Ziconotide is currently only available as an intrathecal medication, and clinical trials were conducted with patients diagnosed with cancer or AIDS (Staats, Yearwood, Charapata, Presley, Wallace, et al., 2004). Although older adults were included in the study, use of this drug should be limited because of numerous and serious side effects.

Opioids

Opioid is a broad term that refers to compounds derived from opium. The term narcotic is often used synonymously with opioids or opiates. However, the term narcotic often has a negative connotation related to illegal use of opiate drugs. Therefore, for the purposes of this chapter, the term opiate or opioid will be used.

Opioids are indicated for moderate to severe acute and persistent pain. These medications can be used safely and effectively in patients. Clinical guidelines have been established by several pain-related professional organizations to facilitate appropriate use of medications for persistent pain (American Academy of Pain Management and the American Pain Society, 1997; AGS, 2002; American Pain Society, 2002; American Society of Anesthesiologists, 1997). Opiates have also shown some efficacy in the treatment of neuropathic pain (Eisenerg, McNicol, & Carr, 2005).

Although clinical practice guidelines are available to guide health care providers, practice guidelines have been used inconsistently (Olsen, Daumit, & Ford, 2006). A recent survey of primary care physicians on opiate prescribing practices showed an increase in opiate prescriptions in the late 1990s that then leveled off in 2000–2001 (Olsen et al., 2006). The increase in opiate prescriptions was attributed to heavy marketing by the makers of Oxycontin® and COX-2 inhibitors, release of practice guidelines, and the emphasis on pain by the Joint Commission on the Accreditation of Health Care Organizations (JCAHO). The recall of two of the COX-2 inhibitors, and investigation of abuse and overdoses related to Oxycontin®, as well as increased physician prosecution related to prescribing opiates has resulted in a leveling of opiate prescriptions written by primary care providers. Some states have adopted intractable pain laws protecting health care providers from legal action if prescribing practices are appropriate. The survey by Olson and colleagues (2006) found that more immediate release opiates were used for persistent pain, which is inconsistent with practice guidelines.

A series of surveys was conducted to examine State Medical Board members' belief about pain, addiction, diversion, and abuse (Gilson, Mauer, & Joranson, 2007). Three surveys were conducted in 1991, 1997, and 2004, which showed a significant improvement in knowledge and attitudes about pain and use of opiates in the treatment of persistent pain. The most recent survey found significant improvement in recognizing that prolonged opiate prescribing is legitimate. In the past, state medical boards determined violation of laws and regulations related to practice and controlled substances. More recently, law enforcement is becoming more active in prosecuting physicians for their prescribing practices. Many state medical boards are adopting policies to facilitate reasonable professional practices related to prescribing controlled substances (Gilson et al., 2007).

There are several classes of opioids. There are full agonists such as morphine, partial agonists such as buprenorphine (used for withdrawal from heroin), mixed agonist-antagonists such as nalbuphine or butorphanol, and antagonists such as naloxone or naltrexone. Opioids target the mu, kappa, and delta receptors. Mu receptors mediate the analgesic effects of morphine and are found in the spinal cord, brain, GI tract, and in the peripheral nervous system. Mixed agonist-antagonist opioids are agonists at kappa receptors and antagonists at mu receptors. Within the mu receptors, there is a degree of variability that accounts for individualized response to opioids.

Opioids have several advantages and disadvantages to their use. All opioids are controlled substances with the exception of tramadol, which is a weak mu receptor opioid and hence not classified as an opiate. Opioid agonists are efficacious, and although most do not have a ceiling effect, in general the higher the dose, the more adverse effects will occur. Most opiates have multiple routes for administration, providing flexibility for patients. The main disadvantage are side effects that can be controlled. Use of multimodal therapies assists in reducing the dose of opiates needed for pain relief. Although opioid agonists are generally safe to use, there is some concern regarding long-term use on hormone and immune function (Dahl, 2005). Hyperalgesia has also been experienced with long-term use of opiates.

Schedule III Medications

Schedule III opioid medications are indicated for mild to moderate pain and have been used for many years. These are oral medications, can be called into pharmacies, and refills are allowed. Many of the opioids in this schedule are combined with aspirin, acetaminophen, or ibuprofen and therefore are limited in their daily dose.

Propoxyphene   Propoxyphene (Darvon®, Darvocet®) has a mild analgesic effect that has the same efficacy of acetaminophen but also has the side effects associated with opiate analgesics. Propoxyphene is on the 2002 Beers list for potentially inappropriate medication use in older adults (Fick et al., 2003). The American Geriatric Society (2002) also cautions against its use due to drug accumulation, neuroexcitatory effects, ataxia, and dizziness that can lead to additional morbidity in older adults.

Codeine   Codeine comes in preparations combined with acetaminophen. Therefore, there is a ceiling of 4,000 mg acetaminophen per day. Codeine is also very constipating and can lead to bowel obstruction if not monitored carefully.

Hydrocodone   Hydrocodone is a short-acting opioid agonist that is use for short-term acute pain or for flare-ups associated with persistent pain. Unless

TABLE 9.4   Hydrocodone Combinations/Formulations

Hydrocodone/Acetaminophen	Hydrocodone/Ibuprofen
2.5/500	7.5/200
5/325	
5/500	
7.5/500	
7.5/750	
10/325	
10/500	
10/650	
10/660	

compounded, hydrocodone is combined with acetaminophen or ibuprofen, thus limiting the daily dosing. The amount of acetaminophen or ibuprofen can be adjusted depending on the formulation prescribed. Hydrocodone has been associated with abuse in part due to the mu2-mediated euphoria and active hydromorphone metabolite (Barkin, Barkin, & Barkin, 2005). Vicodin®, Lortab®, or Lorcet® are common trade names for this medication. Table 9.4 lists the various combinations and dosing formulations available.

Schedule II Opioid Medications

Schedule II opioids can only be prescribed in writing and cannot be called or faxed in to pharmacies. Some mail-order pharmacies request a two or three month prescription, but this needs to be considered very carefully, particularly in the older population. If there is any concern that the patient may have even the slightest cognitive impairment, then the amount dispensed needs to be limited and monitored closely.

Oxycodone   Oxycodone is available in short-acting or extended release oral formulation. Oxycodone as an immediate release medication can be give alone or in combination with 325 or 500 mg acetaminophen. Short-acting formulations are known by trade names such as Percocet®, Endocet®, or Roxicet®. Oxycodone is also available as a solution (15 mg/5 ml). Extended release oxycodone is available as a generic medication or trade name, Oxycontin®. Oxycontin® has been a drug that has significant diversion and abuse. Older individuals tolerate oxycodone and extended release oxycodone fairly well.

Meperidine   Meperidine (Demerol®) is an opioid analgesic that can be administered orally, intramuscularly, or intravenously. One metabolite of meperidine, normeperidine has a long duration of action and stimulates the central nervous system, causing tremors, twitching, and seizures. Meperidine has often been administered with hydroxyzine (Vistaril®) to enhance its effect, although no evidence supports this practice (Dahl, 2005). Hydroxyzine is an anticholinergic drug and associated with orthostatic hypotension and confusion (AGS, 2002). Meperidine also has poor oral absorption. Meperidine should be avoided in older adults and if used should be limited to short procedures. The American Geriatric Society does not recommend its use.

Morphine   Morphine is a pure opioid agonist, and equianalgesic medications are based on morphine concentration. Morphine targets mu receptors, and tolerance can occur, particularly if all the receptors are saturated. Morphine has active metabolites that can accumulate with decreased renal function. It is important to be reminded that extended release formulations of opioid analgesics cannot be crushed or they will become short-acting medications. The exception to this is Kadian®, a 12-hour extended release formulation that can be sprinkled on food. Morphine is available in short-acting tablet, liquid, or sublingual forms. Extended release morphine is available in tablet or capsule form, and formulations last between 8 and 24 hours. Table 9.5 lists the controlled release formulations that are currently available. Controlled release morphine can be administered safely in adults older than age 75. However, doses may be lower than for younger adults (Weil, Ross, Nicholson, & Sasaki, 2007). Morphine can also be administered intravenously and is frequently the drug of choice for patient-controlled analgesia (PCA). Use of morphine in PCA is tolerated well and can provide the provider with information related to analgesic needs. PCA should only be used short-term, and a basal rate should not be used in older adults even if there is no cognitive impairment. Morphine can accumulate and confusion can result.

TABLE 9.5   Extended Release Morphine Formulations

8–12 hours (MS Contin®; Oramorph SR®; Morphine SR)
15, 30, 60, 100 mg doses

>12 hours (Kadian®)
20, 30, 50, 60, 100 mg doses

24 hours (Avinza®)
30, 60, 90, 120 mg doses

Hydromorphone   Hydromorphone (Dilaudid®) is more potent than morphine and is used as an alternative when a patient is allergic to morphine. Hydromorphone can be given intravenously either as an as needed (prn) dose or in PCA. Due to its potency, doses of hydromorphone are small in comparison to morphine. Hydromorphone is available as a short-acting oral medication for break-through pain or flare-ups. A long-acting formulation (Palladone®) was withdrawn from the market due to mortality associated with concurrent alcohol use.

Fentanyl   Fentanyl (Duragesic®) is a lipid soluble, potent opioid agonist. It is dosed in micrograms versus milligrams. It is available for intravenous, transmucosal, buccal, and transdermal administration. Intravenous fentanyl can be used in patient-controlled analgesia but is a more expensive option than morphine or hydromporphone. The transdermal delivery system has a slow onset and duration of 72 hours, making it convenient for patients to administer. Some of the generic formulations appear to have a shorter duration and may need to be changed every 48 rather than 72 hours. Skin irritation where the patch is applied is a common complaint. Transdermal fentanyl is best absorbed with placement on the upper torso, shoulders, or upper back and sites rotated. Absorption is affected by body temperature, subcutaneous fat, and water. Transdermal patches are available in 12.5 mcg, 25 mcg, 50 mcg, 75 mcg and 100 mcg formulations. Fentanyl can also be administered via the transmucosal route (Actiq® lozenges/suckers) or buccal route (Fentora®). The transmucosal or buccal route is useful for painful procedures such as a dressing change or breakthrough pain. The transmucosal dose is not the same for buccal dosing, and consulting a conversion guide is recommended.

Methadone   Methadone is a potent mu opioid-receptor agonist that has existed for a long time, but until recent times it has not been used much for treatment of persistent pain. Methadone is perhaps best known for its use in withdrawal treatment. Interest in methadone has been renewed because it is effective in treating neuropathic pain, and tolerance to this medication is slow to develop. Methadone has a very long half-life, making it not a very good option for older adults, particularly patients with decreased hepatic or renal function. This drug should be avoided in older adults. Prolongation of the QT interval has been demonstrated with methadone use, particularly high doses.

Oxymorphone   Oxymorphone (Opana®, Opana ER®) is an opioid analgesic that has been available for some time, but recently an extended release formulation has become available for the treatment of moderate to severe persistent pain. Packaging labels caution use in older adults because of central nervous system depression. The medication should also be used with caution in patients with mild hepatic impairment or moderate to severe renal impairment. The efficacy of this drug has not been demonstrated on a long-term basis for older adults.

Long-Acting Versus Short-Acting Opioids   Maintaining therapeutic drug levels is a goal for treating acute or persistent pain. Patient-controlled analgesia helps maintain therapeutic drug levels for acute pain. Basal rates are not indicated for older adults due to possible drug accumulation and resulting confusion or somnolence. Long-acting formulations are preferred for treating persistent pain (Vallerand, 2003). Frequent use of short-acting pain medication does not facilitate therapeutic drug levels, and frequent dosing becomes disruptive to one's daily life. If an older adult experiences breakthrough pain prior to the time of the next dose, adjustment to the medication should be considered. Many times providers will prescribe a short-acting medication such as hydrocodone or oxycodone for breakthrough pain. However if this medication is used every day, the patient is basically taking two opioid medications. Short-acting medications should be used only occasionally for exacerbations or flare-ups.

Managing Side Effects of Opioid Medications

Side effects associated with opioid use are predictable and manageable. It is important to anticipate these side effects and take measures to prevent or minimize them. The most common side effects associated with opioid use in older adults include constipation, sedation, psychomotor and cognitive impairment, nausea and vomiting, pruritis, respiratory depression, and delirium.

Constipation is one of the most common side effects of opioid use. Opioids slow motility through the GI system. In addition, older adults do not hydrate themselves adequately. A prophylactic bowel regime should be anticipated. Gentle laxatives such as ducosate and senna are helpful and should be instituted when an opioid is prescribed. Polyethylene glycol (MiraLax®), a tasteless powder and now an over-the-counter medication, may be beneficial. Diet high in fiber is useful and healthy but often not a factor in preventing constipation from opioid use.

Pruritis is another common side effect with intrathecal or epidural opioids. Its mechanism is unclear but may be related to histamine release or involvement of spinal cord receptors. Antihistamines have been helpful with treating the pruritis, but caution must be taken in older adults due to drowsiness experienced from antihistamines. Dosage adjustments may or may not be helpful in reducing the incidence of pruritis.

Sedation associated with opioid use occurs with new therapy or dose increase. Sedation is typically temporary, but if it is prolonged, other causes of sedation should be explored. Older adults need to be aware of sedative effects to prevent falls or other injury.

Nausea and vomiting associated with opioid use is very individual and can be disruptive to one's life. There may be central mechanisms involved in this side effect. Delayed gastric emptying also contributes to nausea and vomiting. Antiemetic medication can be helpful, but once again, adding a medication to counteract a side effect of another drug may not be in the older adult's best interest.

Delirium can occur from opioid use in the older adult population. Decreasing the dose of opioid by 25% or changing to another opioid can be helpful. If reducing the dose of opioid does not clear the delirium, other causes of delirium in the elderly should be considered.

Respiratory depression is a rare side effect of opioid medications when patients are in severe pain. Titration of opioid medication should be slow for older adults. Sedation precedes respiratory depression, so one should be careful to monitor level of arousal.

Short-term opioid use may affect psychomotor skills in any age patient, but particularly older adults. Older adults should refrain from driving or hazardous activity until they are able to function without any psychomotor impairment.

In general, with the exception of constipation, most patients develop a tolerance to side effects of opioids. Side effects often dissipate with time. If side effects persist or develop, switching to another opioid may be helpful. Multimodal therapy may also reduce the dose of the opioid, thus reducing the number of side effects. Patient safety is of utmost importance in prescribing medications.

Long-Term Effects of Opioid Use

The fear of dependence or addiction prevents many patients from obtaining pain relief. The American Pain Society has defined addiction, physical dependence, and tolerance in an effort to educate providers and patients on long-term opioid use for persistent pain.

Addiction is a primary, chronic, neurobiologic disease with genetic, psychosocial, and environmental factors influencing its development and manifestations. It is characterized by behaviors that include one or more of the following: impaired control over drug use, compulsive use, continued use despite harm, and craving.

Physical dependence is a state of adaptation that is manifested by a drug class specific withdrawal syndrome that can be produced by abrupt cessation, rapid dose reduction, decreasing blood level of the drug, and/or administration of an antagonist.

Tolerance is a state of adaptation in which exposure to a drug induces changes that result in a diminution of one or more of the drug's effects over time (http://www.ampainsoc.org/advocacy/opiods2.html).

Tolerance and physical dependence will occur with long-term opioid use. If a person wants to decrease or change medications, the current opioid should be tapered to prevent a withdrawal response.

A patient who is started on opioid therapy for persistent pain should have regularly scheduled visits to evaluate effectiveness of the pain treatment plan and side effects. The provider should specifically ask the older adult exactly how and when they take their pain medication. Use of recreational drugs and alcohol use needs to be assessed at every visit. An opioid medication agreement should be obtained from all patients prior to starting on opioids to insure one provider prescribing and one pharmacy dispensing the drugs. Random toxicology screens are also a part of opioid maintenance.

SUMMARY

Pharmacologic treatment of acute or persistent pain is most efficacious when combining nonpharmacologic and pharmacologic approaches. The use of adjuvant medications along with nonopioid and opioid medications decreases side effects. The cost of medications and therapies must be considered when developing a pain management plan. Side effects of medications need to be anticipated and prevented. The best drug therapy in older adults is achieved with an acceptable balance between symptom control and side effects (Leland, 1999). In general, start doses low, keep regimens simple, and titrate slowly while optimizing function.

REFERENCES

American Academy of Pain Medicine and the American Pain Society. (1997). The use of opioids for the treatment of chronic pain: A consensus statement. *Clinical Journal of Pain, 14,* 6–8.

American Geriatric Society (AGS). (2002). The management of persistent pain in older persons. *Journal of the American Geriatric Society, 50,* S205–S224.

American Pain Society. (2002). *Arthritis pain guideline pain: Guideline for the management of pain in osteoarthritis, rheumatoid arthritis and juvenile chronic arthritis* (2nd ed.). Glenview, IL: American Pain Society.

American Society of Anesthesiologists. (1997). Task force on pain management, chronic pain section: Practice guidelines for chronic pain management. *Anesthesiology, 86,* 995–1004.

Barkin, R. L., Barkin, S. J., & Barkin, D. S. (2005). Perception, assessment, treatment and management of pain in the elderly. *Clinics in Geriatric Medicine, 21,* 465–490.

Dahl, J. (2005). Opioid, non-opioid, adjuvant therapy. Third Annual Comprehensive Pain Board Review, August 2005, Madison, WI.

Eisenberg, E., McNicol, E. D., & Carr, D. B. (2005). Efficacy and safety of opioid agonists in the treatment of neuropathic pain of nonmalignant origin. *Journal of the American Medical Association, 293*(224), 3043–3052.

Fick, D. M., Cooper, J. W., Wade, W., Waller, J. L., Maclean, J. R., & Beers, M. H. (2003). Updating the Beers criteria for potentially inappropriate medication use in older adults. *Archives of Internal Medicine, 163,* 2716–2724.

Gammaitoni, A., Oleka, N., & Gould, E. (2006). Comparison of the efficacy and safety of lidocaine patch 5% versus celecoxib in musculoskeletal conditions: An analysis of a pooled elderly subset. *The Journal of Pain, 7,* S60.

Gana, T. J., Pascual, M. L, Fleming, R. R., Schein, J. R., Janagap, C. C., Xiang, J., et al. (2006). Extended release tramadol in the treatment of osteoarthritis: A multicenter, randomized, double-blind, placebo-controlled clinical trial. *Current Medical Research Opinion, 22*(7), 1391–1401.

Gilson, A. M., Mauer, M. A., & Joranson, D. E. (2007). State medical board members' belief about pain, addition, and diversion and abuse: A changing regulatory environment. *The Journal of Pain, 8*(9), 682–691.

Gloth, F. M. (2001). Pain management in older adults: prevention and treatment. *Journal of the American Geriatric Society, 49,* 188–199.

Goulding, M. R. (2004). Inappropriate medication prescribing for elderly ambulatory care patients. *Archives of Internal Medicine, 164,* 305–312.

Leland, J. Y. (1999). Chronic pain: Primary care treatment of the older patient. *Geriatrics, 54,* 23–37.

Levesque, L. E., Brophy, J. M., & Zhang, B. (2005). The risk for myocardial infarction with cyclooxygenase-2 inhibitors: A population study of elderly adults. *Annals of Internal Medicine, 142*(7), 481–489.

Levesque, L. E., Brophy, J. M., & Zhang, B. (2006). Time variations in the risk of myocardial infarction among elderly users of COX-2 inhibitors. *Canadian Medical Association Journal, 174*(11), 1563–1569.

Olsen, Y., Daumit, G. L., & Ford, D. E. (2006). Opioid prescriptions by U.S. primary care physicians from 1992 to 2001. *The Journal of Pain, 7*(4), 225–235.

Staats, P. S., Yearwood, T., Charapata, S. G., Presley, R. W., Wallace, M. S., Byas-Smith, M., et al. (2004). Intrathecal ziconotide in the treatment of refractory pain in patients with cancer or AIDS. *Journal of the American Medical Association, 29,* 63–70.

Strand, V. (2006) Expectations from patients with rheumatoid arthritis regarding COX-2s: Cutting to the heart of the matter. *Journal of Cardiovascular Pharmacology, 47,* S55–S59.

Vallerand, A. H. (2003). The use of long-acting opioids in chronic pain management. *The Nursing Clinics of North America, 38,* 435–445.

Weil, A., Ross, E., Nicholson, B., & Sasaki, J. (2007). Use of KADIAN for chronic nonmalignant pain in patients > 75 years. *The Journal of Pain, 7*(4), S53.

White, W. B. (2007). Cardiovascular risk, hypertension and NSAIDs. *Current Rheumatology Reports, 9*(1), 36–43.

World Health Organization. (1986). WHO pain ladder. Retrieved January 2, 2008, from http://www.who.int/cancer/palliative/painladder/en/.

Xiang, J., Siccardi, M., Janagap, C., & Vorsanger, G. (2007). Effects of extended-release tramadol on osteoarthritis pain in the elderly. *Pain, 8*(7), S37.

CHAPTER 10

Interventional Therapies

Ann Hoepner

There are many interventions available to reduce acute and persistent pain in older adults. If conservative measures, such as rest, medications, ice, and/or heat, have failed to alleviate discomfort, injection therapy may be the next treatment option, depending on pain location and symptoms. The treatments discussed in this chapter are procedures best performed in a pain specialty clinic, utilizing fluoroscopy in most cases. It is helpful for the health care provider to be familiar with various pain interventions to facilitate the patient's understanding. The following procedures will be discussed: trigger point injections, botox injections, epidural steroid injections, facet blocks, medial branch blocks, and radiofrequency lesioning/neurotomy. Advanced treatment options such as spinal cord stimulation and intrathecal drug delivery will also be addressed.

Before any type of injection therapy is performed, a detailed medical history must be obtained from the patient. Adequate time should be allowed for the older adult to respond to admission questions. A complete medication list is necessary. The use of blood thinners and nonsteroidal anti-inflammatory drugs (NSAIDS), over-the-counter (OTC) and prescribed, must be noted, as some procedures require them to be held prior to injection therapy. For injection therapy to be most beneficial, a definitive diagnosis is needed. Informed consent must be obtained prior to each procedure. Insurance preauthorization may be necessary.

During the patient's procedure, care with positioning is important. Getting on and off narrow procedure tables is sometimes difficult for the older adult. Having sufficient staff to assist and using safety straps are important. Most patients are not comfortable lying on their abdomen, so unnecessary delays should be avoided while they are in this position. Bony prominences are padded to prevent tissue damage. Follow-up care at home should be addressed, as there may be post-procedural extremity weakness, increasing the risk of falling and further injury. Hyperglycemia may occur after corticosteroid injections, particularly in the diabetic older adult. Time frames with ice/heat should be discussed to avoid tissue damage. Easily read written instructions with contact numbers for the patient to refer to when at home should also be provided.

INTERVENTIONAL THERAPIES

Trigger Point Injections

"Musculoskeletal pain is common, frequently under-reported, and inadequately treated in the older adult" (Podichetty, Mazanec, & Biscup, 2003, p. 628). Myofascial pain syndrome is characterized by the presence of trigger points. A trigger point is defined as a hypersensitive knot located in taut muscle. There may be a singular site or multiple points with referred pain that do not follow a dermatomal or nerve root distribution (Alvarez & Rockwell, 2002). The most common locations are the neck, shoulder, and back (Sola & Bonica, 1990). Symptoms associated with myofascial pain/trigger points are constant and localized with palpation of the affected muscle group.

Various treatments for trigger points include biofeedback, pool therapy, physical therapy for myofascial release, and trigger point compression/acupressure. Stretch and strengthening exercises and trigger point injections (TPI) are also helpful treatments.

Trigger point injection therapy involves the injection of various combinations of corticosteroid, local anesthetic, and saline into the trigger point with the intent of relaxing the muscle. Sometimes just the placing of an acupuncture-type needle (dry-needling) into the muscle is enough to relax it. Studies have shown that dry-needling tends to be more uncomfortable, however (Grabois, 2000; McCain, 1994). Complications from trigger point injections are rare and include infection, bleeding, nerve damage, and pneumothorax if injections are over the thoracic area (Travell & Simons, 1983).

Procedure: The clinician in an office setting performs this procedure. Radiology is usually not necessary. Following preparation of the skin, a small gauge needle is inserted into the trigger point palpated by the clinician. This may elicit a twitch response or muscle jump. The medication is then injected into the point and sometimes in fan-like distribution around the site. Ice is applied afterward. Follow-up with physical therapy for stretching and strengthening is crucial. Repeat injection sessions may be necessary.

Botox Injections

Botulism toxin injections may be helpful for the treatment of excessive muscle contraction disorders (Brin & Aoki, 2002). Along with its cosmetic use for facial lines (wrinkles) in the elderly, it can provide relief for blepharospasms, cervical dystonia (torticollis), headaches, myofascial pain syndrome, and spasticity as result of stroke or multiple sclerosis.

Its mechanism of action is inhibition of acetylcholine release resulting in muscle relaxation (Miyamoto, 2004). Once the medication is reconstituted with preservative-free normal saline, the injection procedure is similar to trigger point injections. The dose of botox depends on the patient's weight, and the number and size of muscles to be injected, as well as response to previous injections. Ice is usually not applied afterward. Onset of action is one to three days with peak effect within one to four weeks, and it lasts approximately three to four months (Albany, Cava, Chambers, Childers, Elovic, et al., 2002). Repeat injections are often spaced three months apart. Botulism toxin therapy, in conjunction with physical therapy, provides greatest benefit to the patient (Albany, 2002). Adverse effects from botulism toxin injections may include dysphagia and dry mouth when used for cervical dystonia, and muscle weakness (Albany et al., 2002).

Epidural Steroid Injections

Epidural steroid injection is broad terminology for the injection of corticosteroid mixed with or without local anesthetic into the epidural space, which surrounds the nerves in the spinal canal. A loss-of-resistance syringe is used to advance the spinal needle into the epidural space. It is common practice to use fluoroscopy and nonionic contrast dye with this type of injection treatment. The location of medication placed in the epidural space depends on the pain location, with the rationale of decreasing inflammation to decrease pain. This is a treatment option for patients with generalized spine pain having a radicular component, spinal stenosis, degenerative disk disease, and disk herniation (Elliott, Knox, Renaud, St. Marie, Sharoff, et al., 2002). A series of injections, up to three, may be needed based on response. Wakefield states, "epidural steroid injection seems to be most effective in patients with acute (less than three months' duration) rather than chronic pain" (Wakefield, 1991a, p. 279).

A transforaminal epidural or selective nerve block may be indicated for diagnostic as well as therapeutic reasons. The anti-inflammatory medication is injected at the site of discomfort, in maximum concentration after the nerve root is confirmed with contrast medium and fluoroscopy. This is done to diagnose the radicular pain generator when imaging studies suggest the possibility of more than one area of nerve root compression (Bogduk, 2004; Manchikanti, Staats, Singh, Schultz, Vilims, et al., 2003).

Typically, pain management specialists perform these injections on an outpatient basis. The local anesthetic may provide short-term relief, approximately three to four hours, while the corticosteroid may take three to seven days before relief is noted (Wakefield, 1991a). Risks include infection, bleeding, post-dural puncture headache, and nerve damage. Diabetic patients may experience hyperglycemia requiring additional insulin (Abram, 2000).

For pain relief near end of life, neurolytic blocks may be indicated. If the patient responded well to a local anesthetic trial, alcohol or phenol is injected for longer symptom relief (Joseph & deLeon-Casasola, 2000; Wakefield, 1991c).

Facet Joint Injections/Medial Branch Blocks

Zygapophysial or facet joints are the small pairs of joints between the articular processes of the vertebrae (Bogduk & Twomey, 1991; Wakefield, 1991b). Facet joints are injected for diagnostic as well as therapeutic reasons. Corticosteroid with local anesthetic is injected under fluoroscopic guidance. Nonionic contrast dye may be used. Symptom relief during the local anesthetic phase provides diagnostic information. The steroid may effectively settle down pain due to inflammation as a therapeutic effect.

There are two nerves that innervate each zygapophysial joint. These medial branch nerves carry signals, including pain, away from the spine and control small muscles of the spine, not sensation or motor function of the arms and legs (Baker, 2006). Blocking the medial branches with local anesthetic will provide further diagnostic information as to location of the pain generator. Medial branch block injections are performed with fluoroscopic guidance as well as nonionic contrast dye. Local anesthetic only is usually injected. Patients monitor their response, doing usual activities, during the time frame of the anesthetic's effectiveness. If the medial branch block is effective, then radiofrequency medial branch neurotomy or radiofrequency lesioning may provide the patient a longer sense of relief.

Patients who present with localized neck pain radiating to the occiput or shoulder areas or back and hip pain radiating across the buttocks to the thighs may have degeneration of facet joints. These patients have increased pain with extension of their neck or back. Tenderness upon palpation over the facet joint is present. There may be radiographic confirmation of degeneration of the facet joints (Hogan, 2000a, 2000b). Adverse effects from facet injections or medial branch blocks are similar to the risks from epidural injection therapy.

Radiofrequency Neurotomy/Lesioning

If the patient experienced short-term relief from the zygapophysial joint injection and relief during the local anesthetic phase of the medial branch block, the patient may be a candidate for percutaneous radiofrequency medial branch neurotomy or radiofrequency lesioning. This procedure involves use of special electrodes placed by the pain management specialist, using fluoroscopy. Positioning is the same as for the facet/medial branch blocks. The radiofrequency lesioning takes longer due to the sensory and motor testing that is done at each site to further confirm proper electrode placement. The local anesthetic is then injected in most cases. The lesioning is performed using high-frequency electrical currents to coagulate the nerve tissue (Bogduk, 2004). The duration of the current is 60–180 seconds per site.

The rationale behind the radiofrequency lesioning is to disrupt the pain signals from the joint. There is irritation caused by the lesioning; therefore, most patients do not experience symptom relief until two to three weeks post-procedure. Nerves do regenerate over time, sometimes necessitating repeating the procedure (Baker, 2004). Risks of this procedure are the same as previous injection therapies. Complications are rare and include numbness or muscle paralysis (Elliott et al., 2002).

ADVANCED TREATMENT OPTIONS

Advanced treatment options such as spinal cord stimulation (SCS) and intrathecal infusion pumps (i.e. drug administration systems or DAS) are possible options if conservative measures and injection therapies for nonmalignant chronic pain and cancer pain have been tried without success. Some pain management or neurology services are equipped with staff and resources for these procedures. Ongoing care with qualified personnel is crucial. Both treatment modalities involve a trial process to determine if it is an effective treatment prior to surgical implantation of the devices. Insurance preauthorization is needed due to initial and ongoing cost of the treatment. However, studies have shown that over time the therapy pays for itself because the cost of oral or transdermal medications as well as office and emergency department visits are reduced (Manchikanti et al., 2003; Deere, Chapple, Classen, Javery, Stoker, et al., 2004; Kumar, Kelly, & Pirlot, 2001; Kumar, Hunter, & Demeria, 2002). Most insurance companies follow Medicare guidelines requiring a physical assessment as well as psychological assessment stating why the treatment modality is appropriate for the patient (Van Dorsten, 2006).

Spinal Cord Stimulation (SCS)

Spinal cord stimulation (SCS) involves the use of low-intensity electrical impulses to trigger the nerve fibers along the spinal cord. Figure 10.1 provides an illustration of this technology. According to Melzak and Wall, stimulating these nerves causes the pain message sent to the brain to be diminished or blocked (Wall & Melzack, 1994). However, the exact mechanism of actions

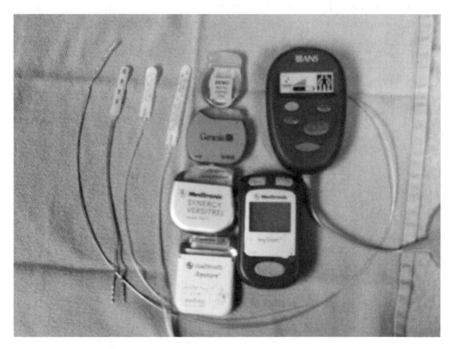

FIGURE 10.1   Spinal Cord Stimulation (SCS)
(Spinal Cord Stimulator Equipment: Left to right, Leads, Power Sources, Patient Programmers)

continues to be explored (Linderoth & Foreman, 2006). The patient's sharp, shooting, shock-type pains are perceived as "pleasant parasthesia" with use of SCS. Patients use various words to describe this feeling, such as tingling and massaging.

SCS may be a viable treatment option for patients with neuropathic pain as a result of failed back/neck surgery syndrome, complex regional pain syndrome, arachnoiditis, chronic intractable angina pain, and pain from peripheral vascular disease (Goldstein & Gilbert, 2005; Manchikanti et al., 2003). SCS has also been helpful for patients with phantom limb pain.

Contraindications for this treatment modality include patients with untreated psychosis or major depression, patients with untreated alcohol or drug habituation, patients with unrealistic expectations of the device, and patients who do not obtain effective pain relief during the trial or are unable to operate the equipment. Patients with coagulopathy may not be candidates if they are unable to safely be off their anticoagulant during the trial and surgery. Patients with cardiac pacemakers/defibrillators may also be excluded, depending on the equipment brand. Patients with SCS are unable to have MRIs post-implantation because of the metal electrodes interfering with the diagnostic test.

There are several key advantages with SCS, including patient control over pain in a nonpharmalogical method. Most times, the patient will use SCS in place of short-acting pain medication. The use of adjuvant medications such as gabapentin, pregabalin, and duloxetine will continue due to the relief they provide for neuropathetic pain. However, dosages may be able to be decreased. The patient has the ability to turn on the stimulator when he/she is uncomfortable and make adjustments with different programs and sensations, depending on how the pain is at that point in time. Treatment is individualized in regards to timing and duration of SCS usage. SCS is considered a reversible procedure. The system can be removed without any structural changes to the body.

SCS implantation is a lengthy process and follow-up with knowledgeable support staff is important. Some facilities utilize the equipment representatives for assistance in programming the stimulators under the supervision of the physician. Other facilities have specially trained staff. Some equipment companies, Medtronic and Advanced Neuromodulation Systems (ANS), offer ongoing education and technical support for facilities interested in offering this type of treatment to their patients.

Patient and family education is very important. During the education process, assessments regarding cognitive level, mobility, skin integrity, and presence of sensory impairments are made. The physician decides which equipment to use based on those assessments.

After insurance preauthorization, and the physical and behavioral health assessments are obtained, the patient undergoes the SCS trial for a short time period and actually "test drives" the equipment to see if the spinal cord stimulation provides effective pain relief for him or her. The equipment used is similar to if not the same as in the permanent implantation. The battery source is external during the trial. This may be an outpatient or inpatient procedure, depending on medical coverage and the facility.

The SCS trial is considered a success if there is effective pain relief. Some facilities require 50–75% reduction in pain as their criteria. There should be an increase in function and the ability to run the equipment. Expectations of spinal cord stimulation should be realistic; 100% pain relief is not obtainable. SCS is a treatment option to aid in pain management, not a cure. SCS is not an appropriate treatment option for patients who feel the stimulation in painful areas but do not experience sufficient/pleasant relief.

Permanent Implantation

All components are placed under the skin for permanent implantation of the SCS system. The lead(s) is placed, as in the trial, with patient participation if a permanent lead was not used initially. The X-ray from the trial lead placement is used as a guide as well as the pain diagram and fluoroscopy. Depending on where the power source is placed, extensions may be used. These are tunneled under the skin and connected to both the lead and the power source. Common locations for the power source are the upper buttocks and lower abdomen.

The patient's pain pattern, the need for one or two leads, the number of electrodes needed to provide pain relief, and time usage are all factors the pain specialist assesses when determining the type of power source. Body mass and size of power source are also factored in. The SCS systems that are powered by radio frequency require an antenna to be placed on the skin over the implanted receiver. This small, circular paddle is connected to the power source, which is also the patient's programmer. Skin integrity must be monitored, as the antenna is held in place by adhesive. The rechargeable battery SCS systems require a recharging unit belted over the battery site for 30–90 minutes weekly/monthly. Location of the power source is important, as the patient may not be flexible enough to place the antenna/recharging unit on the upper buttock area.

The patient has a programmer with the ability to turn the stimulation on and off, switch to different programs, and make adjustments within that program to individualize the sensation to fit how he is feeling at that point in time. The three main parameters are amplitude, pulse width, and rate or frequency. Amplitude is the intensity or strength of the stimulation similar to the volume on a radio. This is measured in volts or milliamps. Pulse width is the duration of electrical pulse and is measured in microseconds. As pulse width is increased, the area of stimulation widens, much like the waves created when a rock is thrown in water. The rate or frequency is the number of pulses per second and is measured in hertz. Patients describe sensations as smooth or thumping when the rate is adjusted.

Some programmers are more user-friendly for arthritic hands. Some programmers have symbols instead of writing and use raised buttons to aid with visually impaired patients. When the clinician is programming the stimulator, the cognitive level of the patient needs to be kept in mind, as there is the ability for numerous stimulation programs. Some patients turn their stimulator on and adjust only the amplitude setting. The goal of programming is to cover the patient's pain as simply as possible. If the programming is too complicated, the patient may not use the stimulator system at all.

Follow-up surgical care is important to monitor incision healing as well as stimulation effectiveness. Post-operative X-rays are taken and compared to the intra-operative ones. The location of the lead(s) directs the clinician with programming of the electrodes. It often takes a number of sessions to find adequate pain relief programs. Figure 10.2 illustrates two types of permanent spinal cord stimulators currently available.

Adverse Events

Following SCS implantation, the patient needs to be followed closely for any surgical complication. Some surgical complications include bleeding, nerve damage, and infection. Bleeding may occur during or after the surgery; bleeding in the epidural space may lead to nerve damage. An infection may lead to meningitis or an epidural abscess, requiring the total system removal. A dural-puncture headache, injury to the spinal cord, and incisional seroma collection of fluid in the battery pocket are also adverse effects of implantation (Medtronic Synchromed II Programable Infusion System Clinical Reference Guide, 2004). System-related complications include lead migration and equipment failure (Manchikanti et al., 2003). The patient needs to be aware of these complications and notify appropriate health care providers immediately.

Drug Administration Systems

Intrathecal drug therapy is another advanced treatment modality (Winkelmuller, Burchiel, & Buyten, 1999). It involves medication delivery from either

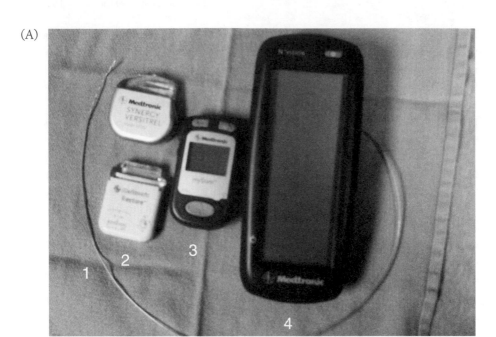

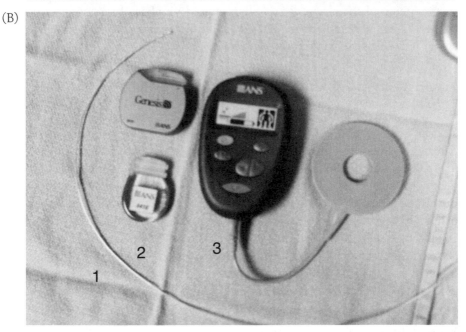

FIGURE 10.2   (A) Medtronic Equipment; (B) ANS Equipment
Left to right: (1) leads, (2) power source, (3) patient programmer, (4) clinical programmer

a programmable or nonprogrammable pump via a catheter into the cerebral spinal fluid. The drug administration system (DAS) is totally implanted under the skin, with the patient returning to the clinic for routine medication refills.

Indications for an implantable drug delivery system include intractable pain of malignant or nonmalignant origin, inadequate pain relief and/or intolerable side effects from systemic medication, and severe spasticity of spinal origin (Gianino, York, & Paice, 1996). Contraindications for this treatment would be patients with untreated psychosis/major depression, patients with untreated alcohol or drug habituation, and patients with unrealistic expectations of the device. Patients with coagulopathy may not be candidates if they are unable to safely be off their anticoagulant for the epidural trial and surgery.

Pumps are implanted in patients with malignant or chronic nonmalignant pain. Pain pumps work by inhibiting the release of certain neurotransmitters, thereby blocking the pain signal before it reaches the level of perception (Gianino et al., 1996). This takes place in the dorsal horn, which contains a high density of opioid receptors.

Intrathecal drug therapy may be indicated in patients who develop tolerance to the point where high doses of systemic opioid medication are needed for pain relief. The higher the levels of opiates, the greater the risk of side effects experienced by the patient. Intrathecal opioid medication can be given in much smaller doses because it is being delivered in close proximity to the pain receptors in the spinal cord (Manchikanti et al., 2003). Side effects such as nausea, vomiting, pruritus, and sedation may occur but usually subside within 24–48 hours.

Some elderly patients have difficulty tolerating oral pain medication. They are extremely sensitive to any type of opioid medication—oral or transdermal—and yet have uncontrolled pain. These patients should also be considered as possible candidates, as intrathecal medication delivery may be better tolerated (Roberts, Finch, Goucke, & Price, 2001; Winkelmuller & Winkelmuller, 1996).

Some patients with spinal cord injuries, multiple sclerosis, or cerebral palsy have spasticity problems that are better controlled by the intrathecal delivery of baclofen. Baclofen pumps work by increasing the amount of the neurotransmitter gamma-aminobutyric acid (GABA) that induces muscle relaxation, which leads to a decrease in spasticity.

Some of the key advantages of DAS include the fact that the medication is being delivered to the site of action in the spinal cord in steady amounts. The constant levels maintain more even control of pain or spasticity depending on the medication used. Eliminating the sensation of "peaks and valleys" that sometimes occurs with oral medications results in a more consistent, effective pain/spasticity relief. Smaller doses are possible because the medication does not have to cross the blood-brain barrier and is at the site of action. The lower dosing may result in reduced side effects (Kumar et al., 2001). Figure 10.3 illustrates one type of reservoir for the DAS system.

The process of DAS is lengthy and should not be taken lightly. It requires time and commitment from both patient and care provider. Patient and family education is essential. The DAS trial occurs before permanent implantation

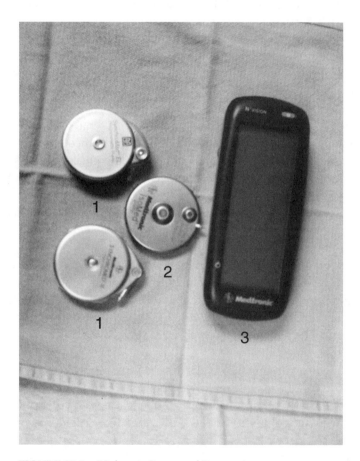

FIGURE 10.3   Medtronic Pumps and Programmer
(1) Programmable; or (2) nonprogrammable pump; (3) clinician
programmer.

to determine if the medication will be effective with minimum side effects. It is performed with the same medication that will be used in the permanent pump. Morphine and baclofen (Lioresal) are the FDA-approved agents for intrathecal delivery via an implanted pump. There are many other alternate agents that clinicians choose to use based on individualized patient needs and clinic philosophy (Bennett, Deer, et al., 2000; Bennett, Serafini, et al., 2000). Hydromorphone (Diluadid) is an example of another common medication used for intrathecal delivery.

Implantation

Prior to permanent implantation of the DAS, a screening trial is conducted. Thee screening can be conducted a variety of ways, via bolus injection or continuously with a catheter connected to an external pump. The clinician determines which method to use based on the patient's medical status, whether or not the patient has hardware from previous surgeries, and caregiver support. The bolus method involves morphine injected intrathecally or epidurally. The ratio of intrathecal dose to epidural dose is 1:10. Common starting morphine amounts are 0.5–1.0 mg intrathecally or 5–10 mg epidurally (Pasero, Portenoy, & McCaffery, 1999). If the trial medication is baclofen (Lioresal), it must be injected intrathecally, because it does not cross the meningeal membrane (Gianino et al., 1996). The starting bolus amount is 50 mcg, but this must be individualized based on the patient's current medications. Functional and spasticity assessments are made prior to bolus injection and every hour for approximately eight hours by a physical therapist.

A continuous infusion of medication trial most closely mimics the permanent system implantation. This involves placement of a catheter into the epidural or intrathecal space. The epidural catheter placement is similar to spinal cord stimulator lead placement. Some physicians tunnel the catheter a short distance from the insertion site to further decrease risk of infection and/or catheter migration. The catheter is connected to an external pump and medication bag. Some facilities require patients to be off all their opioid medications for the trial. Other facilities use a titration process in which pump medication is increased while the patient decreases oral/transdermal doses. Either way, the patient returns for frequent office visits for medication adjustments and pain assessments.

The trial is considered successful if there has been more effective pain relief with minimum side effects and a decrease in oral/transdermal pain medications. It is a positive baclofen trial if spasticity/stiffness is diminished and noticeable by the patient and physical therapist with minimum side effects.

Surgery for permanent implantation may be performed under general or monitored anesthesia. The intrathecal catheter is placed under fluoroscopy and tunneled to the pump, which is usually placed in the lower abdomen. Care is taken regarding the positioning of the pump so it does not rest by the bladder or catch on the ribs. The patient must have sufficient body mass to handle the hockey puck-sized pump.

There are two types of pumps, programmable and nonprogrammable. The programmable pump is battery-powered and lasts five to seven years then must be replaced. The clinician programmer is able to get information from the pump as well as make dosage adjustments in rate and timing of medication doses. The nonprogrammable pump runs on freon gas and does not need replacing. It has a factory-set flow rate that is delivered on a daily basis. The patient will need a refill with a change in concentration to adjust the medication dose.

All the pumps have a reservoir that holds the liquid medication. Most of the pumps have access ports directly to the catheter and cerebral spinal fluid (CSF). This is helpful if there is a concern regarding the integrity of the catheter. After the medication is removed, contrast medium can be injected through this port and the system checked under fluoroscopy for leaks or disconnects. Some facilities do myelograms through the access port, eliminating the risk of dural-puncture headaches.

Medication dosing is an individualized event. The expectations of the patient, his family, and the medical staff must be consistent, appropriate, and verified frequently. Each clinic has its own philosophy regarding opioid medications. The predominant thought for persistent nonmalignant pain is that the pump medication is delivering the long-acting medication, negating the need for oral long-acting opioids. There may be a need for short-acting, breakthrough medication. The propensity for the breakthrough medication to become a daily requirement instead of on an as-needed basis is something that requires frequent discussion and review of nonpharmalogical pain-relieving methods with the patient and caregivers.

Adverse Events

As the intrathecal catheter is placed, there needs to be CSF reflux confirming proper placement of the catheter. Sometimes CSF leaks around the catheter, resulting in a dural puncture or "spinal" headache. There have been occasions where the CSF has actually tracked around the tunneled catheter and pooled in the pump pocket, creating a fistula. A purse-string suture around the catheter insertion site may help. Neurosurgical repair may be necessary to re-place the catheter in a different location and repair the leak if this complication occurs.

Bleeding may occur and collect in the pump pocket, forming a hematoma. Special attention to hemostasis during the pocket formation will help prevent a hematoma. Serous fluid may also collect to the point where fluid aspiration is necessary. The use of an abdominal binder postoperatively is a preventative measure.

Infection is a rare, but very serious complication that may lead to total drug delivery system (DAS) removal. An intraspinal abscess may lead to spinal cord compression, sepsis, or paralysis. Preoperative antibiotics and meticulous care with skin and equipment preparation are crucial.

Both of the advanced treatment options (SCS and DAS) have provided the right patient population with adequate pain relief (Deer et al., 2004; Kumar et al., 2002; Kumar et al., 2001; Paice, Penn, & Shott, 2006) and with improved quality of life. They are treatment options that need careful consideration with ongoing patient and family education and follow-up. A total patient assessment including physical, psychological, and social-economic status is warranted.

SUMMARY

Interventional pain therapies have provided longer-term relief of symptoms for many patients. The treatment options outlined in this chapter are tolerated well by older adults. Advanced treatment options open a new avenue for continuous administration of medication to relieve pain or control spasticity.

REFERENCES

Abram, S. (2000). Epidural steroid injections. In S. Abram & J. Haddox (Eds.), *The pain clinic manual* (2nd ed., pp. 393–396). Philadelphia: Lippincott Williams & Wilkins.

Albany, K. (2002). Physical and occupational therapy considerations in adult patients receiving botulinum toxin injections for spasticity. In N. Mayer & D. Simpson (Eds.), *Spasticity: Etiology, evaluation, management and the role of botulism toxin.* Produced by WE MOVE, World Wide Education and Awareness for Movement Disorders.

Albany, K., Cava, T., Chambers, H., Childers, M., Elovic, E., Esquenazi, A., et al. (2002). Dosing, administration, and a treatment algorithm for use of botulinum toxin type A for adult-onset muscle overactivity in patients with an upper moto-neuron lesion. In N. Mayer & D. Simpson (Eds.), *Spasticity: Etiology, evaluation, management and the role of botulism toxin.* Produced by WE MOVE, World Wide Education and Awareness for Movement Disorders.

Alvarez, D., & Rockwell, P. (2002, February 15). Trigger points: Diagnosis and management. *American Family Physician, 65*(4), 653–660., F Baker, R. (2004). Radio-frequency neurotomy for facet and sacroiliac joint pain. Retrieved November 1, 2006, from http://www.spine-health.com/topics/conserv/radio/radio01.html.

Baker, R. (2006). Medial branch nerve blocks. Retrieved November 1, 2006, from http://www.spine-health.com/topics/diag/block01.html.

Bennett, G., Deer, T., Du Pen, S., Rauck, R., Yaksh, T., & Hassenbusch, S. J. (2000). Future directions in management of pain by intraspinal drug delivery. *Journal of Pain and Symptom Management, 20,* 44–50.

Bennett, G., Serafini, M., Burchiel, K., Buchser, E., Classen, A., Deer, T., et al. (2000). Evidence-based review of literature on intrathecal delivery of pain medicine. *Journal of Pain and Symptom Management, 20,* S12–S31.

Bogduk, N. (2004). *Practice guidelines for spinal diagnostic and treatment procedures.* San Francisco: International Spine Intervention Society.

Bogduk, N., & Twomey, L. (1991). *Clinical anatomy of the lumbar spine* (2nd ed.). Melbourne: Churchill Livingstone.

Brin, M., & Aoki, R. (2002). Botulism toxin type A: Pharmacology. In N. Mayer & D. Simpson (Eds.), *Spasticity: Etiology, evaluation, management and the role of botulism toxin.* Produced by WE MOVE, World Wide Education and Awareness for Movement Disorders.

Deer, T., Chapple, I., Classen, A., Javery, K., Stoker, V., Tonder, L., et al. (2004). Intrathecal drug delivery for treatment of chronic low back pain: Report from the national outcomes registry for low back pain. *Pain Medicine, 5,* 6–13.

Elliott, J., Knox, K., Renaud, E., St. Marie, B., Sharoff, L., Swift, M., et al. (2002). Chronic pain management. In B. St. Marie (Ed.), *Core curriculum for pain management nursing* (pp. 273–347). Philadelphia: W.B. Saunders.

Gianino, J. M., York, M. M., & Paice, J. A. (1996). *Intrathecal drug therapy for spasticity and pain.* New York: Springer.

Goldstein, L., & Gilbert, S. (2005). Neurostimulation in chronic pain patients. *Practical Pain Management, 5,* 30–31.

Grabois, M. (2000). Myofascial pain syndrome. In S. Abram & J. Haddox (Eds.), *The pain clinic manual* (2nd ed., pp. 167–176). Philadelphia: Lippincott Williams & Wilkins.

Hogan, Q. (2000a). Back pain and radiculopathy. In S. Abram & J. Haddox (Eds.), *The pain clinic manual* (2nd ed., pp. 157–166). Philadelphia: Lippincott Williams & Wilkins.

Hogan, Q. (2000b). Diagnostic and prognostic nerve blocks. In S. Abram & J. Haddox (Eds.), *The pain clinic manual* (2nd ed., pp. 61–67). Philadelphia: Lippincott Williams & Wilkins.

Joseph, P., & deLeon-Casasola, O. (2000). Neurolytic blocks and other neuroablative procedures for cancer pain. In S. Abram & J. Haddox (Eds.), *The pain clinic manual* (2nd ed., pp. 375–389). Philadelphia: Lippincott Williams & Wilkins.

Kumar, K., Hunter, G., & Demeria, D. (2002). Treatment of chronic pain using intrathecal drug therapy compared with conventional pain therapies: A cost-effectiveness analysis. *Journal of Neurosurgery, 97,* 803–810.

Kumar, K., Kelly, M., & Pirlot, T. (2001). Continuous intrathecal morphine treatment for chronic pain of nonmalignant etiology: Long-term benefits and efficacy. *Surgical Neurology, 55,* 79–86.

Linderoth, B., & Foreman, R. (2006). Mechanisms of spinal cord stimulation in painful syndromes: Role of animal models. *Pain Medicine, 7,* S14–S26.

Manchikanti, L., Staats, P., Singh, V., Schultz, D., Vilims, B., Jasper, J., et al. (2003). Evidence-based practice guidelines for interventional techniques in the management of chronic spinal pain. *Pain Physician, 6,* 3–81.

McCain, G. (1994). Fibromyalgia and myofascial pain syndromes. In P. Wall & R. Melzack (Eds.), *Textbook of pain* (3rd ed., pp. 475–493). New York: Churchill Livingstone.

Medtronic synchromed II programmable infusion system clinical reference guide. (2004, April). Minneapolis, MN: Medtronic Corporation.

Miyamoto, M. (2004). Agents affecting neuromuscular transmission. In C. Craig & R. Stitzel (Eds.), *Modern pharmacology with clinical applications* (6th ed., pp. 338–347). Baltimore: Lippincott Williams & Wilkins.

Paice, J. A., Penn, R. D., & Shott, S. (1996). Intraspinal morphine for chronic pain: A retrospective, multicenter study. *Journal of Pain and Symptom Management, 11,* 71–80.

Pasero, C., Portenoy, R., & McCaffery, M. (1999). Opioid analgesics. In M. McCaffery & C. Pasero (Eds.), *Pain clinic manual* (2nd ed., pp. 674–710). Philadelphia: Mosby.

Podichetty, V., Mazanec, D., & Biscup, R. (2003). Chronic non-malignant musculoskeletal pain in older adults: Clinical issues and opioid intervention. *Postgraduate Medical Journal, 79*(937), 627–633.

Roberts, L. J., Finch, P. M., Goucke, C. R., & Price, L. M. (2001). Outcome of intrathecal opioids in chronic non-cancer pain. *European Journal of Pain, 5,* 353–361.

Sola, A., & Bonica, J. (1990). Myofascial pain syndromes. In J. Bonica (Ed.), *The management of pain* (2nd ed. pp. 352–366). Philadelphia: Lea & Febiger.

Travell, J., & Simons, D. (1983). *Myofascial pain and dysfunction the trigger point manual.* Baltimore: Williams & Wilkins.

Vallerand, A. H. (2003). The use of long-acting opioids in chronic pain management. *The Nursing Clinics of North America, 38,* 435–445.

Van Dorsten, B. (2006). Psychological considerations in preparing patients for implant procedures. *Pain Medicine, 7,* S47–S57.

Wakefield, C. (1991a). Epidural steroids. In C. Warfield (Ed.), *Manual of pain management* (pp. 276–280). Philadelphia: J. B. Lippincott.

Wakefield, C. (1991b). Facet injections. In C. Warfield (Ed.), *Manual of pain management* (pp. 281–285). Philadelphia: J. B. Lippincott.

Wakefield, C. (1991c). Nerve blocks. In C. Warfield (Ed.), *Manual of pain management* (pp. 271–275). Philadelphia: J. B. Lippincott.

Wall, P., & Melzack, R. (1994) *Textbook of pain*. New York: Churchill Livingstone.

Winkelmuller, M., & Winkelmuller, W. (1996). Long-term effects of continuous intrathecal opioid treatment in chronic pain of nonmalignant etiology. *Journal of Neurosurgery, 85*, 458–467.

Winkelmuller, W., Burchiel, K., & Van Buyten, J. P. (1999). Intrathecal opioid therapy for pain: Efficacy and outcomes. *Neuromodulation, 2*, 67–76.

CHAPTER 11

Adaptations to Improve Function

Michele Komp-Webb

Adapting the home environment is a very important component in managing persistent pain. Unfortunately there is very little research available about improving safety and function in homes of those with persistent pain. Most research is based on home evaluations and treatment interventions related to falls. Home modification recommendations are generally similar for each group based on the shared trait of being elderly. Because most individuals, those who fall or those with pain, consider home a safe environment, they may not realize how long-used habits will negatively affect their symptoms and safety. Medication, therapy, and educational interventions may be negated when an individual with persistent pain returns home and engages in activities they have not identified as pain-generating or unsafe.

Home visits should be considered for all hospitalized older adults (Cumming et al., 1999) and those with persistent pain whether or not they have been hospitalized. A study by Cumming and colleagues (2001) notes that of 178 homes visited, modifications were recommended in 150. Follow-up visits one year after the initial visit revealed only 52% compliance. The researchers concluded that most older adults do not believe that adapting their home environment will reduce their falls.

Note: The author acknowledges Sara Sipple, OTR, CHT, for her assistance in writing this chapter.

The same can be said of home modifications to reduce pain. Two studies identified that environmental factors, as opposed to medication or health issues, are more likely to be involved in falls at home in active individuals than in those who are frail (Northridge, Nevitt, Kelsey, & Link, 1995; Speechley & Tenetti, 1991). Intervention for any individual at risk for injury should include muscle strengthening and balance retraining prescribed by a trained health professional, identification of home hazards and modifications that are professionally prescribed, and withdrawal of psychotropic drugs (Gillespie et al., 2001). It is of interest to note that Stevens and colleagues (2001), performed a randomized controlled trial that concluded that a one-time intervention program of education, hazard assessment, and home modifications to reduce fall hazards in the homes of healthy older people is not an effective strategy for the prevention of falls in seniors. This relates to the 52% compliance rate identified previously. For a home assessment to be beneficial, follow-up by a health care professional, several months after the home changes have been made, should be provided.

As the population of geriatric individuals increases, home modifications will be critical in assisting this group to "age in place," regardless if they have persistent pain, a history of falls, or other medical conditions. A study by Bayer and Harper (2000) concluded that 80% of individuals over the age of 50 want to age in their homes. They will be able to do so comfortably and safely utilizing home and activity adaptations. Assessments should not be limited to just the home but include travel, leisure activities, functional activities, and locomotion. A needs assessment should be conducted with each individual and should identify specific problems or needs, solutions, how to implement the solutions, training of the individual, and evaluation of outcomes. Training of family members or support staff is also important. Although data collected at the time of discharge is helpful in determining the necessary changes needed to return home, an in-home assessment of instrumental activities of daily living (IADLS) remains key to understanding the complex skills required to live alone at home (Lysack & Neufeld, 2003).

THE ROLE OF OCCUPATIONAL THERAPISTS AND ASSISTANTS

Occupational therapists (OTR, Occupational Therapist, Registered) and occupational therapy assistants (COTA, Certified Occupational Therapy Assistants) are certified health care professionals that are trained specifically to assist individuals in returning to work, home, bathing, dressing, and leisure activities. They are often the health professional of choice to conduct and follow up on home assessments. Cumming and colleagues (1999) concluded that home visits performed by an occupational therapist may also lead to changes in behavior that enable older people to live more safely in both the home and external environment.

Many OTs undergo specialized training to become certified hand therapists (CHT). These experts receive additional training emphasizing custom splint fabrication for the purpose of pain relief, immobilization, restraint, support of a body part, joint protection, proper positioning, proper alignment of bony and soft tissues, and promotion of proper healing of bony or soft tissue injury. For example if an individual with chronic pain has a difficult time placing weight through the wrist and hands to propel a walker, occupational therapists can fabricate an appropriate splint to transfer the force to another area of the upper extremity, such as the forearm, or alter the force through the wrist and hand.

Occupational therapists may accept referrals from physicians, dentists, podiatrists, advanced practice nurses, chiropractors, optometrists, physician assistants, psychologists, or other health care providers. Reimbursement is extremely variable for services, splinting, and assistive devices.

ADAPTING THE ENVIRONMENT

Following is a list of activities and situations with solutions to reduce pain and improve function in older adults. This list is a guideline and is not intended to be inclusive.

Home

There are various rooms and activities that occur in the home that can be easily adapted to facilitate ease of movement and reduce pain in older adults. Various modifications in each room or activity will be discussed briefly. Table 11.1 provides a worksheet for the older person or family member to adapt their home to improve safety and reduce pain.

Kitchen

Utensils with built-up or weighted handles, rocker knives, angled utensils or swivel utensils will decrease force on the hands and fingers. This is particularly useful for older adults with arthritis. Jar and bottle openers, can tab pullers, electric can openers, studded cutting boards, electric appliances, weighted cups, and plates with edges will make meal preparation and eating easier.

TABLE 11.1 Home Modification for Improved Function Checklist

Activity/Location	Need Identified	Solution Implemented	Follow-up: 6 and 12 months
Kitchen:			
Utensils: handle build-up, weighted handles or order special items such as rocker knives, swivel or angled utensils			
Flatware: dishes with edges, weighted or covered cups			
Other: jar/can openers, can tab pullers, electrical appliances, studded cutting board			
Appliances: Toaster oven to replace large oven.			
Easy-to-use timer for stove for safety			
General: Commonly used items placed shoulder to hip height, easy-open cupboard handles, removal of throw rugs			
Bathroom:			
Bathing: bath mitt, long handled sponge, terrycloth robe for drying, bath chair, non-slip bath mat			
Grooming: long-handled comb, chair			
Other: raised toilet seat, grab bars, throw rugs, pillbox			
Living Room:			
Raised furniture, removal of throw rugs, lift chair, touch lights, large-button remote, coffee table with lift top			
Bedroom:			
Bed on blocks, portable grab bar on bed, lightweight blankets, blanket stand at foot of bed			
Hallways:			
Handrails, removal of throw rugs, lighting			

194

TABLE 11.1 (Continued)

Activity/Location	Need Identified	Solution Implemented	Follow-up: 6 and 12 months
General all rooms: Touch light switches, adequate lighting, enlarged lamp switches, removal of throw rugs, door knob grippers/convert to levers, easy to carry portable phone, ramps into house, built-up keys			
Dressing: Sock aides, button hooks, elastic shoe laces, long-handled shoe horns, zipper pulls, Velcro closings, elastic waist bands, pull-on over head clothing, slip-on shoes, lightweight clothing to decrease pressure on sensitive skin, appropriate, well-fitting footwear.			
Cleaning: Cleaning products on each level, eliminate throw rugs, self-propelled vacuum, long-handled cleaning products, feather dusters, elevated washer/dryer			
Leisure: Book holders, card holders, spring-loaded scissors, prop sewing/book on lap with pillow			
Personal general: Know the effects of medication, make sure eyewear fits appropriately, especially vari-focal glasses, don't perform activities when fatigued, delegate tasks, pace activities, warm up before arduous tasks, alternate repetitive activities with restful activities, use larger muscle groups when able			

(Continued)

195

TABLE 11.1 (Continued)

Activity/Location	Need Identified	Solution Implemented	Follow-up: 6 and 12 months
Gardening: Long-handled or ergonomic tools, easy-to-pull garden carts that act as a bench, carpenter's aprons with multiple pockets (portable phone), wrap tool handles with foam grips			
Travel: *Vehicles*: can be modified with door-open assist, adjustable seats, steering wheel covers, seatbelt handles, heated back rests and seats; extreme modifications are available to accommodate many handicaps. Taller vehicles are easier to enter/exit than cars. Plan to stop and rest frequently during long trips. *Plane/train*: call ahead for assistance to and around the terminal. Aisle seats to allow mobility during the trip, luggage on wheels, compression garments during flight.			
Shopping: Four- or three-wheeled (rollator) walkers with a basket and/or seat, use of motorized cart if available, long-handled bags carried over the shoulder, backpacks, wheeled luggage			
Ambulation and locomotion: Canes, walkers, crutches, lofstrand crutches, two-wheeled walkers, standard walkers, rollator walker, scooters, wheelchairs, electric wheelchairs, modified hand or forearm rests			

Commonly used kitchen items should be placed in cupboards from shoulder to hip height to decrease reaching and bending.

Bathroom

The use of a bath mitt instead of a washcloth will decrease the work on fingers. Using a long handled sponge will decrease the amount of bending and reaching during bathing. Bath chairs will decrease energy expenditure. Using a terrycloth robe to dry instead of towel drying by hand will conserve energy. Raised toilet seats decrease the effort of transferring to and from the seat. Grab bars are an excellent safety feature. Placing a chair in the bathroom for shaving and hair styling will also conserve energy. Long handled brushes and combs are available to assist with grooming.

Living Room

Raising furniture on wooden blocks will make sitting and rising easier. Lift chairs will assist in conserving energy and decreasing pain. Touch lights and large-button remotes are available to decrease motion in painful hands. Coffee tables with lift tops will promote improved posture, decreased pain, and decreased effort when reading and eating.

Hallways

Installing handrails and eliminating throw rugs will improve safety. Adequate lighting is also essential.

Bedrooms

Placing beds on blocks and/or adding portable handrails will make it easier to get in and out the bed. Lightweight comforters make turning in bed less difficult. Blanket stands can be placed at the foot of the bed to lift up sheets from painful feet and also make turning easier. Appropriate beds and mattresses are specific to each individual and one type will not be beneficial for everyone, despite what the manufacturers report.

Dressing

Sock aides, button hooks, elastic shoe laces, long handled shoe horns, zipper pulls, Velcro closings, elastic waist bands, and clothing that pulls on over the head will all make dressing easier and less painful. Lightweight sports clothing made of nylon blends will decrease friction over skin for individuals with shingles or allodynia.

Cleaning

Cleaning products should be kept on each level of the home to decrease the need for stair climbing and carrying. Using a self-propelling vacuum with a push motion instead of pulling will decrease energy expenditure and strain on the low back. There are many long-handled cleaning products available. Feather dusters and other dusting aides with handles will decrease strain on hands compared to a cloth and spray. Front-loading washers and dryers can be placed on blocks to improve body mechanics.

Leisure

Book holders, card holders, and spring-loaded scissors are available to decrease hand/arm strain and assist in decreasing pain. When reading or sewing, stress to the arms and neck can be decreased by propping the book/item on a pillow on the lap.

General

Wall switches can be converted to those that engage with a tap. Lamp switches can be enlarged with a piece of plastic that fits over the existing switch. All throw rugs should be removed from high-traffic areas to decrease falls and cleaning effort. Doorknob grippers can be installed or knobs can be converted to levers. Ramps can be installed outside the home, and chair lifts or small elevators are available for inside the home. Portable phones on each level of the house will improve safety. When possible, phones should have clasps to attach to clothing for easier carrying. Cabinet handles and knobs can be easily changed to allow for easier gripping and opening. Built-up keys are also available for individuals with decreased dexterity due to pain. Pillboxes with large, easy-open lids are helpful in reducing medication administration errors and loss of medication.

Gardening

Gardening provides leisure and relaxation for many older individuals. Many elderly people believe that they cannot enjoy their gardens due to painful conditions. Long-handled tools are available to reduce bending or kneeling.

Easy-to-pull garden carts are available and equipped to carry tools and be used as a sitting bench. Carpenter's aprons with multiple pockets can carry many tools and a portable phone. Tool handles can be wrapped with foam grips to improve comfort and decrease hand strain. Many garden tools have bent handles to improve ergonomics. Water supplies should be close to the garden to minimize unnecessary steps.

Travel

Older persons can become isolated because they restrict their travel. Short or long trips are often too painful and disruptive to their routines. Many older adults rely on family member to drive or provide transportation. Younger family members are likely to stop less often, leading to long periods of time with minimal joint or muscle movement and resulting is stiffness and discomfort.

Vehicles

Most vehicles can be modified with door open assist, adjustable seats, steering wheel covers, seatbelt handles, heated back rests and seats, and/or massaging seat covers to improve comfort and ease of driving. Vans, trucks, and SUVs will be easier to enter than a car. Simple modifications such as a kitchen chair cushion may elevate the car seat enough to decrease pain getting out of a car. Extreme modifications to any vehicle are available to assist individuals' special needs but are costly. Plans to stop and rest frequently on long trips will decrease back and neck stress.

Planes/Trains

Most airports and depots have assistance available for traveling to and around the terminals. Calling ahead and making arrangements to be greeted with a wheelchair or cart can improve traveling comfort. Aisle seating is preferable for standing and stretching during long trips. Luggage on wheels or luggage carts will decrease strain on the entire body. For plane travel, compression garments for the upper and/or lower extremities may decrease the pain associated with static, dependent positions, and cabin pressure changes.

Shopping

Four- or three-wheeled walkers with seats and baskets will allow for frequent rests and provide carrying assistance. Many stores offer motorized carts.

Long-handled bags carried over the shoulder or paper bags carried close to the body are easier on the arms and back than plastic bags carried at the side. Backpacks are an excellent option as long as they are not overfilled or heavy.

Ambulation and Locomotion

There are many assistive devices available to improve mobility and safety. Standard equipment includes canes, crutches, lofstrand crutches, two-wheeled walkers, traditional walkers, four-wheeled walkers, scooters, wheelchairs, motorized wheelchairs, and rollator walkers (a walker with a seat and a basket). Modifications to standard equipment can be made to improve comfort. Armrests can be installed on walkers so weight bearing is done through the forearms and not the hands. Hand grips can be fitted to canes and walkers. Placing tennis balls on the back legs of traditional walkers or two-wheeled walkers allows for easier propulsion but maintains safety.

Interestingly, the more stable assistive device is not always the safest. An evaluation of several devices should be performed by a health care professional to determine the most appropriate device.

GENERAL GUIDELINES FOR ACTIVITIES AND TASKS

First and foremost, any tasks that are painful or exhausting should be delegated. Gentle warm-up stretches or activities should be performed prior to longer or more arduous tasks. Walking around a room several times is adequate to improve circulation and get joints and muscles ready to work. Each task should be broken down into small increments, with rest stops planned. Repetitive activities should be paced or alternated with other activities or rests. Larger muscle groups and joints should be used when possible; for example, one should use the shoulder to open a heavy door and not the hand.

RESOURCES

Sources for adaptive supplies can be found at local drug stores, large retail chains, churches, hardware stores, free clinics, loan closets, and through home care agencies and adult day care facilities. Consulting with occupational therapists, physical therapists, social workers, or other health care professionals will enable individuals to secure devices and locate resources.

A list of resources that may be helpful to providers in adapting environments or obtaining equipment to reduce pain in older persons is included at the end of this chapter. The list is not inclusive. Knowing community as well as other resources is a key in facilitating the older person to adapt their environment and reduce their pain.

REIMBURSEMENT

Reimbursement is variable, and the lack of reimbursement can result in an older person choosing not to purchase an adaptable piece of equipment. Medicare guidelines change frequently and other insurance coverage is extremely variable. Local suppliers may offer discounts for those using Medicare. Payment assistance may be available locally through county agencies. It is strongly suggested that all payors be contacted prior to purchase of any assistive device. Caution against bias is recommended, as Lysack and Neufeld (2003) identified that publicly insured patients received fewer home modification recommendations compared to privately insured patients.

REFERENCES

Bayer, A. H., & Harper, L. (2000). Fixing to stay: A national survey on housing and home modification issues. American Association of Retired Persons. Retrieved January 3, 2008, from http://www.aarp.org/research/reference/publicopinions/aresearch-import-783.html.

Cumming, R., Thomas, M., Szonly, G., Salkeld, G., O'Neill, E., Westbury, C., et al. (1999). Home visits by occupational therapists for assessment and modification of environmental hazards: A randomized trial of fall prevention. *Journal of the American Geriatric Society, 47*(12), 1397–1402.

Cumming, R., Thomas, M., Szonly, G., Frampton, G., Salked, G., & Clemson, L.. (2001). Adherence to occupational therapist recommendations for home modifications for falls prevention. *American Journal of Occupational Therapy, 55*(6), 641–648.

Gillespie, L. D., Gillespie, W. J., Robertson, M. C., Lamb, S. E., Cumming, R. G., & Rowe, B. H.. (2001). Interventions for preventing falls in elderly people. *Cochrane Database System Review, 3,* CD000340.

Lysack, C. L., & Neufeld, S. (2003). Occupational therapist home evaluations: Inequalities but doing the best we can? *American Journal of Occupational Therapy, 57*(4), 369–379.

Northridge, M. E., Nevitt, M. C., Kelsey, J. L., & Link, B..(1995). Home hazards and falls in the elderly: The role of health and functional status. *American Journal of Public Health, 85,* 505–515.

Speechley, M., & Tenetti, M. (1991). Falls and injuries in frail and vigorous community elderly persons. *Journal of American Geriatric Society, 39,* 46–52.
Stevens, M., Holmen, C. D., Bennett, N., & de Klerk, N. (2001). Preventing falls in
older people: Outcome evaluation of a randomized controlled trial. *Journal of
American Geriatric Society, 49*(11), 1448–1455.

List of National Resources

American Chronic Pain Association
PO Box 850
Rocklin, CA 95677
800.533.3231
www.theacpa.org

American Geriatrics Society
The Empire State Building
350 5th Avenue South
New York, NY 10118
212.308.1414
www.theamericangeriatricssociety.org

American Occupational Therapist Association
4720 Montgomery Lane
Bethesda, MD 20814-3425
301.652. AOTA (2682)
www.aota.org

American Pain Society
4700 West Lake Avenue
Glenview, IL 60025-1485
877.734.8758
www.ampainsoc.org

American Physical Therapy Association
1111 North Fairfax Street
Alexandria, VA 22314-1488
800.999.APTA (2782)
www.apta.org
http://headtotoe.apta.org

Mayo Clinic
200 1st Street Southwest
Rochester, MN 55905
507.284.2511
www.mayoclinic.com

National Resource Center on Supported Housing and Home Modification
Andrus Gerontology Center
University of Southern California
3715 McClintock Avenue
Los Angeles, CA 90089-0191
213.740.1364
www.homemods.org

National Arthritis Foundation
3400 Peachtree Road Northeast
Atlanta, GA 30326
State and local chapters established
www.arthritis.org

National Institute of Arthritis and Musculoskeletal and Skin Diseases
1 AMS Circle
Bethesda, MD 20892-2190
301.496.4000
www.niams.nih.gov

National Institute of Dental and Crainiofacial Resources
(This is the primary National Institute of Health organization for
pain research)
National Institute of Health
Bethesda, MD 20892-3675
800.624.BONE (2663)
www.nidcv.nig.gov

National Institute of Health
Osteoporoses and related Bone Diseases
National Resource Center
2 AMS Circle
Bethesda, MD 20892-3675
www.osteo.org

National Institute of Health Pain Consortium
9000 Rockville Pike
Bethesda, MD 20892-3675
301.496.4000
www.painconsortium.nih.gov

National Institute of Neurological Disorders and Stroke
(Pain page available)
PO Box 5801
Bethesda, MD 20824
800.352.9424
www.ninds.nih.gov

CHAPTER 12

Challenges to Treating Older Adults Living With Persistent Pain

Michaelene P. Jansen

Like any chronic illness, living with persistent pain takes a toll on an individual's personal, social, physiological, mental, and financial state. No matter how effective one's coping skills, there are sequelae related to persistent pain that affect behavior and function. The earlier the pain is managed and function restored, the fewer the negative consequences for that person. How to best manage pain in older adults continues to challenge health care providers.

The intent of this chapter is to examine some of the barriers that exist in attempting to manage persistent pain in older adults. Numerous references have addressed the under-treatment of pain in older adults (Ferrell, Novy, Sullivan, Banja, Dubois, et al., 2001). Health care providers are challenged by economic, social, and regulatory issues. Ethical dilemmas related to pain treatment in older adults continue to play a role in effectively managing pain in older adults. There is no disagreement that the health care system has an obligation to provide comfort and pain management for older adults (AGS, 2002). There remains, however, a discrepancy between setting realistic goals for older adults in persistent pain and meeting those goals.

BARRIERS

Several major barriers exist that prevent older adults from obtaining and maintaining adequate pain relief. A survey of health care professionals including physicians, nurses, pharmacists, and social workers was conducted by Ferrell and colleagues (2001). The investigators identified several factors that contribute to ethical dilemmas in pain management that can also be identified as barriers to adequate pain management. These barriers include inappropriate pain management; barriers to care; interactions and conflicts among families, patients, or providers; and regulatory issues.

Inappropriate Pain Management

Many providers admit to under-treating persistent nonmalignant pain. There are several contributing factors that lead to inappropriate pain management. Some providers have acknowledged that their own judgments and biases play into the treatment plan for persistent nonmalignant pain (Ferrell et al., 2001). Studies have demonstrated that medications including patient-controlled analgesia can be safely administered in older adults (Gagliese, Jackson, Ritvo, Wowk, & Katz, 2000).

Other factors that contributed to inappropriate pain management identified by Ferrell and colleagues (2001) include fear of substance abuse, violation of pain contracts, unwillingness to prescribe analgesics in older adults based solely on age, and over-use of invasive procedures. Older adults are often hesitant to take analgesic medications, especially opiate analgesic medications, due to fear of dependency. This fear is often reinforced by family members and providers, leading to inadequate pain management.

Gender may also influence prescribing practices. Goulding (2004) found that older women were at higher risk for analgesic drugs being prescribed inappropriately than older men. Gender roles have shown to influence sensitivity to pain and may not be adequately evaluated in the assessment and management of pain in older adults (Campbell, Edwards, Hastie, & Filligim, 2007). One study found women to have a stronger relationship between disability and mood compared to men. This study suggests that men relate disability directly to pain, whereas women tend to view their pain associated with their disability in negative terms (Hirsh, Waxenberg, Atchison, Germillion, & Robinson, 2006).

Economic Barriers

Economic barriers continue to hinder adequate pain treatment for patients and health care providers. For example, reimbursement agencies deny reimbursement for a consult and procedure on the same day. This can lead to delay in treatment, particularly for a patient who travels a great distance to be treated. Delay in treatment can influence other aspects of an older adult's life such independence, mobility, and quality of life. Many insurance plans and pharmacy formularies do not allow coverage for certain medications or procedures. Many hours are spent by the patient and health care provider obtaining prior authorization, which also contributes to delay in treatment. In obtaining prior authorization, many older adults need to "fail" on a preferred pharmaceutical agent before the desired medication is approved. "Preferred" drugs may not be the drug of choice for the older adult due to undesirable side effects. Pharmacists have also expressed frustration with out-of-date formularies that limit access to newer drugs and therapies because they are "too expensive" or "have not proven effective" (Ferrell et al., 2001, p. 178). Schatman (2007) expresses his frustration that the refusal for third-party reimbursement of multidisciplinary pain centers has led to closure of these centers and increased reliance on opiates and interventional means to manage pain.

A qualitative study interviewing executives from six health maintenance organizations found that there was a lack of an integrated, multidisciplinary approach to pain management and a lack of data related to cost effectiveness of various pharmacologic and nonpharmacologic treatments (Pellino, Gordon, & Dhal, 2006). There exists an obvious need for further research in this area, especially as it relates to older adults.

Social Barriers

Many social issues influence pain perception and may not be addressed adequately during pain assessment of older adults. Chapter 5 addresses the intricate relationship between sleep and pain as well as pain and sleep. Edwards and colleagues (2007) found that less than 6 hours or more than 10 hours of sleep will affect perception of pain. It is important to examine sleep as a contributing factor, because pain as well as pain analgesics can disrupt sleep. Some of the treatments for sleep allow for long periods of deep sleep, and many older adults complain of stiffness and difficulty with joint movement due to the lack of movement during their sleep.

Social support has been associated with perceived severity of persistent pain. Decreased social support has been identified as a factor contributing to catastrophizing (Buenaver, Edwards, & Haythornthwaite, 2007). Catastrophizing is a cognitive and emotional response magnifying pain and pain-related stimuli. Feelings of helplessness and negativism accompany catastrophizing. The concept of catastrophizing is an important variable to address in persistent pain (Edwards, Bingham, Bathon, & Haythornwaite, 2006). Psychosocial and pharmacologic treatment can help limit catastrophizing, but in older adults, any addition of medication puts the older adult at higher risk for drug interactions.

Social factors may also limit an older person's ability to participate in treatment. Transportation, inclement weather (particularly ice), and cost are just a few factors identified that may hinder access to care and treatment (Austrian, Kerns, & Reid, 2005). For example, transportation to and from appointments or therapy may need to be arranged by public transportation or family member. If an older person resides in a rural community without public or elderly transportation and has no family in close proximity, it may be difficult to arrange appointments. Many older persons are unable to afford a membership at a local pool or fitness center or do not have local access to these facilities for therapy or exercise.

Regulatory or Policy Barriers

Several professional standards or guidelines exist for treating pain in older adults (AGS, 2002; Wisconsin Medical Society Task Force on Pain Management, 2004; Institute for Clinical Systems Improvement, 2007). These guidelines, based on clinical evidence and research, assist health care professionals in providing standards of care in treating pain. The guidelines are dynamic and have scheduled reviews to provide revisions and updates based on new clinical evidence. However, guidelines are only as good as they are implemented and utilized. All providers need to be aware of the guidelines and resources available related to management of pain in older adults.

The role of drug enforcement is having an increased effect on providers' willingness to provide adequate analgesic medications, particularly if it involves controlled substances. Prosecution of physicians related to opioid analgesic use has made many providers hesitant to provide ongoing opioids for persistent pain. As a result, many providers refer their patients to regional pain centers. Referrals to pain centers may or may not be feasible or geographically possible for many older adults. Frequent follow-up and monitoring is critical in managing persistent pain in the older population. The use of pain contracts should be initiated with all patients receiving ongoing pain analgesics for patient and provider safety.

The Joint Commission on the Accreditation of Health Care Organizations (JCAHO) has helped improve assessment and management of pain in health care organizations by including adequate documentation of pain assessment and follow-up after intervention as part of their criteria for accreditation. This requirement has encouraged hospitals, and medical, nursing, and allied health schools to offer educational programs or curricular content on pain.

Legislative efforts have also been critical in appropriating funding for pain research. The U.S. Congress declared 2000–2010 as the Decade of Pain Control and Research (HR 1863), providing funding for laboratory and clinical research. Legislation such as the National Pain Care Policy Act of 2007 intends to improve pain care research, education, training, access, outreach, and care. The legislation also provides measures to increase public awareness and improve professional training as well as establish a Pain Consortium at the National Institutes of Health (National Library of Congress, 2007).

Ethics

The most frequently encountered dilemmas in health care relate to inadequate treatment of pain. It is interesting that nursing literature addresses pain management as an ethical issue more frequently than medical literature (Ferrell et al., 2001). One of the difficulties noted in addressing adequate pain management is that currently a patient's self-report of pain is a major part of pain assessment. The response to the self-report of pain is what continues to be the variable that leads to debate. In some expert opinions, fully accepting an older adult's report of pain may lead to too much liberal use of opiates or may lead to undertreatment, in other viewpoints (Ferrell et al., 2001). A provider may often be forced to decide between drug control standards and pain control standards.

Multidisciplinary task forces on ethics in pain management would be beneficial to address the many ethical issues and dilemmas that exist in relation to pain in the older adult. It is anticipated that health care providers will encounter more ethical decisions and issues related to pain in older adults on a more frequent basis as that population increases. Policy statements and ethical codes by professional organizations will help strengthen the quality of care provided to older adults with pain (Ferrell et al., 2001).

EDUCATION

Education related to pain and pain management cannot be overemphasized. There has been great progress in pain awareness over the past decade, particularly because this past decade has been declared the Decade of Pain Control and Research. However, there is still much more that needs to be done in terms of education for patients, families, health professionals, and communities.

Professional Education

Health care professional education, including of physicians, advanced practitioners, nurses, pharmacists, physical therapists, and occupational therapists needs to have more formal content on mechanisms of pain transmission, modulation, and pharmacologic and nonpharmacologic strategies. Understanding the relationship of sleep, depression, and affective distress to pain is critical in formulating a comprehensive plan for treating pain. In addition, content specific to the older adult needs to be integrated, including but not limited to geropharmacotherapeutics, physiology of aging, and functional assessment of the older adult, as well as assessment of cognitive functioning.

Patient Education

Patients and families require ongoing education regarding pain conditions prevalent in older adults, overall treatment plans, and awareness of potential adverse effects or consequences of treatment choices. Treatment plans that are simple and easy to follow can minimize error and margins of interpretation. It is best if treatment plans are written, in large or bold print with the patient's name and date identified on the plan. Table 12.1 provides an example of an instructional treatment plan.

Clarification of the treatment plan should be reviewed at each appointment. Adjustments and modifications should be dated or a new plan with

TABLE 12.1 Sample Treatment Plan

Name: Sample Patient	Date: Current date
Diagnosis: Osteoarthritis; postherpetic neuralgia	

7:00 A.M.	Stretching exercises upon arising
	Apply lidocaine 5% patch to area of pain related to shingles
	Take morning pain medications
	    Extra-strength acetaminophen (500 mg) 1–2 tablets
	    Gabapentin 300 mg

9:00 A.M.	Morning exercises (pool exercises or walking)
12:00 noon	Gabapentin 300 mg. May take with lunch
4:00 P.M.	Stretching/balance/gait exercises
5:00 P.M.	Gabapentin 300 mg. May take with supper
Bedtime	Remove lidocaine 5% patch Extra strength acetaminophen 500 mg 1–2 tablets if needed

Note: Acetaminophen is not contraindicated in this patient example.

the date of the revisions should be given to the patient. Frequent monitoring and communication are keys in limiting prescribing or administration errors (Gloth, 2001).

Community Education

Misperceptions regarding pain, particularly persistent pain, are common in community settings. Community programs increasing awareness of causes, treatment, and options for pain management are well received. The greater the understanding within a community, the greater the acceptance and support for patients, particularly older adults with persistent pain. Social support has been found to be an important variable in the perception of pain (Buenaver et al., 2007).

FUTURE RESEARCH AND TREATMENT

As pain research continues to have priority in federal research agendas, it is anticipated that our understanding of pain will increase. For example, there appear to be some significant advances in using ion channel blockers to modulate pain. Animal studies have demonstrated the possibility of selectively blocking the excitability of primary sensory nociceptors by using a lidocaine derivative and capsaicin, which opens up the cell membrane to allow the blocking agent in (Binshtok, Bean, & Woolf, 2007). This form of treatment is unique because it uses an ion channel to deliver medication.

Recent advances in understanding the mechanisms involved in neuropathic pain have resulted in newer, more effective pain medications with fewer side effects. There is some belief that neuropathic pain has some features of a neuroimmune disorder, opening the door for treatment options involving immunosuppression and blocking neuronal signals (Scholz & Woolf, 2007).

Reexamining old concepts and theories may also provide new insight and ways of understanding, treating, and modulating pain. Goldberg (2007) suggests that the biopsychosocial model may not be adequate and suggests that pain specialists and researchers reexamine the old Cartesian model of pain. Mathematical modeling has provided insight into molecular, cellular, and neural networks related to brain plasticity and its role in persistent pain (Britton & Skevington, 1996).

The role of genetics may also provide some insight into pain perception and sensitivity to pain. Genetic predictors of acute and persistent pain are still in their infancy (Edwards, 2006b). Over the next several years and decades, the identification of genetic, biologic, and environmental predictors will be paramount in adequately assessing, treating, and understanding pain.

SUMMARY

It has been well established that pain-related disability is a major contributing factor in the quality of life in older adults. Pain is often under-treated in older adults. Many myths exist regarding pain perception and sensitivity in older adults (Weiner, 2005). Pain severity plays a role in the disability of older adults compared to younger adults (Edwards, 2006a). The quality of the pain rather than intensity of the pain may be more important in older adults than younger adults (Gagliese & Melzack, 2003). Pain management plans should be individualized and age-related. Barriers, unfortunately, still exist in preventing adequate pain relief in older adults. Access to care, social constraints, regulatory mandates, and inadequate education are a few of the barriers that still need to be overcome. Health care providers are encouraged to meet the challenge of adequately treating and managing older adults experiencing pain with dignity and quality of care.

REFERENCES

American Geriatric Society. (2002). The management of persistent pain in older adults. *Journal of the American Geriatric Society, 50,* S205–S224.

Austrian, J. S., Kerns, R. D., & Reid, M. C. (2005). Perceived barriers to trying self-management approaches for chronic pain in older persons. *Journal of the American Geriatric Society, 53*(5), 856–861.

Binshtok, A. M., Bean, B. P., & Woolf, C. J. (2007). Inhibition of nociceptors by TRPV1-medicated entry of impermeant sodium channel blockers. *Nature, 449*(7162), 607–610.

Britton, N. F., & Skevington, S. M. (1996). On the mathematical modeling of pain. *Neurochemical Research, 21,* 1133–1140.

Buenaver, L. F., Edwards, R. R., & Haythornthwaite, J. A. (2007). Pain-related catastrophizing and perceived social responses: Inter-relationships in the context of chronic pain. *Pain, 127,* 234–242.

Campbell, C., Edwards, R., Hastie, B., & Filligim, R. (2007). Age and sex differences in pain perception: The role of gender role stereotypes. *The Journal of Pain, 8,* S60.

Edwards, R. R. (2006a). Age differences in the correlates of physical functioning in patients with chronic pain. *Journal of Aging and Health, 18*(1), 56–69.

Edwards, R. R. (2006b). Genetic predictors of acute and chronic pain. *Current Opinion in Rheumatology, 86,* 411–417.

Edwards, R. R., Bingham, C. O., Bathon, J., & Haythornwaite, J. A. (2006). Catastrophizing and pain in arthritis, fibromyalgia and other rheumatic diseases. *Arthritis and Rheumatology, 55*(2), 325–332.

Edwards, R., Haythronthwaite, J., Klick, B., & Smith, M. (2007). Disturbances of sleep contribute to next-day pain report in the general population. *The Journal of Pain, 8,* S52.

Ferrell, B. R., Novy, D., Sullivan, M. D, Banja, J., Dubois, M. Y., Gitlin, M. C., et al. (2001). Ethical dilemmas in pain management. *The Journal of Pain, 2*(3), 171–180.

Gagliese, L., & Melzack, M. (2003). Age-related differences in the qualities but not the intensity of chronic pain. *Pain, 104*(3), 597–608.

Gagliese, L., Jackson, M., Ritvo, P., Wowk, A., & Katz, J. (2000). Age is not an impediment to effective use of patient-controlled analgesia by surgical patients. *Anesthesiology, 93*(3), 601–610.

Gloth, F. M. (2001). Pain management in older adults: Prevention and treatment. *Journal of the American Geriatrics Society, 49,* 188–199.

Goldberg, J. S. (2007). Revisiting the Cartesian model of pain. *Medical Hypotheses.* doi:10.1016/mety.2007.08.01.4.

Goulding, M. R. (2004). Inappropriate medication prescribing for elderly ambulatory care patients. *Archives of Internal Medicine, 164,* 305–312.

Hirsh, A. T., Waxenberg, L. B., Atchison, J. W., Germillion, H. A., & Robinson, M. E. (2006). Evidence for sex differences in the relationships of pain, mood and disability. *The Journal of Pain, 7,* 592–601.

Institute for Clinical Systems Improvement (ICSI). (2007). Assessment and management of chronic pain. Bloomington, MN: Author.

National Library of Congress (2007). National Pain Care Policy Act 2007. Retrieved January 3, 2008, from http://thomas.loc.gov/beta/billView.jsp?&exact=false&pb Summary=false&searchBSS=false&searchCmte=false&searchCR=false& searchCurrent=false&searchMulti=false&searchOtr=false&searchPN=false &searchPrevious=false&searchTre=false&swr=true&versions=true&con gress=110&viewurl=billView.jsp&action=text&currDoc=1&currentPage=1& numHits=1&k2dockey=%2Fprd%2Fk2%2Fbills%2Fxml%2F110%2Fh2994. ih.xml%40billmerge&action=text.

Pellino, T. A., Gordon, D. B., & Dahl, J. L. (2006). The Wisconsin's Pain Initiative's review of Wisconsin's managed care climate for pain management: Opportunities for improvement. *Wisconsin Medical Journal, 105,* 27–32.

Schatman, M. (2007). Our ethical obligation to treat chronic pain and suffering: A response to the growth of technophilism in chronic pain management. *The Journal of Pain, 8,* S86.

Scholz, J., & Woolf, C. J. (2007). The neuropathic pain triad: Neurons, immune cells and glia. *Nature Neuroscience, 10*(11), 1361–1368.

Weiner, D. K. (2005). Pain in older adults. *National Pain Foundation*. Retrieved January 3, 2008, from www.nationalpainfoundation.org/MyTreatment/News_Pain andtheOlderAdult.asp.

Wisconsin Medical Society Task Force on Pain Management. (2004). Guidelines for the assessment and management of chronic pain. *Wisconsin Medical Journal, 103*(3), 1–43.

Index

Evidence-Based Geriatric Nursing Protocols for Best Practice

Third Edition

Elizabeth Capezuti, PhD, RN, FAAN
DeAnne Zwicker, MS, APRN, BC
Mathy Mezey, EdD, RN, FAAN
Terry T. Fulmer, PhD, RN, FAAN, Editors
Deanna Gray-Miceli, DNSc, APRN,
Associate Editor
Malvina Kluger, Managing Editor

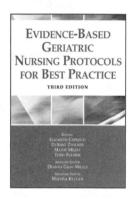

"This third edition holds the promise of bringing yet another level of depth and sophistication to understanding the best practices for assessment, interventions, and anticipated outcomes in our care of older adults. **Evidence-Based Geriatric Nursing Protocols for Best Practice** *is intended to bring the most current, evidence-based protocols known to experts in geriatric nursing to the audience of students, both graduate and undergraduate, practitioners at the staff level from novice to expert, clinicians in specialty roles (educators, care managers, and advanced practice nurses), and nursing leaders of all levels."*
—from the Preface by **Susan Bowar-Ferres,** PhD, RN, CNAA-BC
Senior Vice President & Chief Nursing Officer
New York University Hospitals Center

This is the third, thoroughly revised and updated edition of the book formerly entitled **Geriatric Nursing Protocols for Best Practice.** The protocols address key clinical conditions and circumstances likely to be encountered by a hospital nurse caring for older adults. They represent "best practices" for acute care of the elderly as developed by nursing experts around the country as part of the *Hartford Foundation's Nurses Improving Care to the Hospitalized Elderly project (NICHE).*

This third edition includes 17 revised and updated chapters and more than 15 new topics including critical care, diabetes, hydration, oral health care, palliative care, and substance abuse.

2007 · 736pp · 978-0-8261-1103-6 · hardcover

11 West 42nd Street, New York, NY 10036-8002 • Fax: 212-941-7842
Order Toll-Free: 877-687-7476 • Order Online: www.springerpub.com

SPRINGER PUBLISHING COMPANY

Complementary and Integrative Medicine in Pain Management

Editors: Michael I. Weintraub, MD, FACP, FAAN
Ravinder Mamtani, MBBS, MD, MSc
Marc S. Micozzi, MD, PhD

Pain is the most common complaint amongst all patients seeking care from all types of health practitioners. It is estimated that 40% of patient visits to health care practitioners are for the management of pain.

The problem of pain and other functional complaints is an ever larger proportion of the practice of integrative medicine. Complementary and alternative medical modalities have much to offer in managing pain and functional complaints, as well as presenting new and unique perspectives on the phenomenon of pain.

This book is also unique in taking into account cultural, historical and social factors in pain and pain management. While not a topic in itself (with the exception of the introductory chapter) it is a perspective that infuses all the topics of the book.

Special Features
- Contributions from national experts providing unique benefits of knowledge and experience on each topic
- Extensive information on remedies and treatment modalities, such as acupuncture, herbal medicine, homeopathy and massage, manual and manipulative therapies
- Evidence based approach with discussions of the advantages and limitations of each type of treatment based upon current clinical studies
- Provides added options for treatment and management of chronic pain and neurological disorders
- Treatment options for neurologic conditions, including migraine and tension headache, stress, dementia, Parkinson's disease, and other common conditions

2008 · 480pp · 978-0-8261-2874-4 · hardcover

11 West 42nd Street, New York, NY 10036-8002 • Fax: 212-941-7842
Order Toll-Free: 877-687-7476 • Order Online: www.springerpub.com

Mindfulness-Based Elder Care

A CAM Model for Frail Elders and Their Caregivers

Lucia McBee, LCSW, MPH

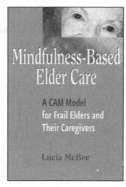

"She shares with us her gold—the conception, trial and error implementation, and initial scientific investigation of a new, educationally-oriented treatment approach that she has named mindfulness-based elder care (MBEC)."

—from the Foreword by **Saki Santorelli,** EdD, MA, Associate Professor of Medicine, Executive Director, Center for Mindfulness in Medicine, Health Care, and Society, University of Massachusetts Medical School

Drawing on years of experience as a geriatric social worker and mindfulness-based stress reduction practitioner, the author has taken Jon Kabat-Zinn's *Mindfulness-Based Stress Reduction* program and adapted it to the particular needs of elders, their families, and professional caregivers. Mindfulness practices focus on abilities, rather than disabilities, in order to provide paths to the inner strengths and resources that we all possess. McBee's **Mindfulness-Based Elder Care** conveys the benefits of mindfulness through meditation, gentle yoga, massage, aromatherapy, humor and other creative therapies, accessibly, to this special population. She provides clear, concise instructions for her program, as well as a wealth of anecdotal and experiential exercises to help readers at all levels of experience. Hers is the first book to fully explore the value of mindfulness models for frail elders and their caregivers.

Features of this groundbreaking volume include
- Valuable tips for establishing programs to address each population's specific needs and restrictions
- Design for short classes or 8-week courses
- Detailed experiential exercSoftcoverises for the reader
- Numerous case studies
- Clear, easy-to-follow instructions for elders and caregivers at all levels

2008 · 240pp · 978-0-8261-1511-9 · softcover

11 West 42nd Street, New York, NY 10036-8002 • Fax: 212-941-7842
Order Toll-Free: 877-687-7476 • Order Online: www.springerpub.com

Palliative Care Nursing

2nd Edition
Quality Care to the End of Life

Marianne LaPorte Matzo, PhD, RN, GNP, CS
Deborah Witt Sherman, PhD, RN, ANP, CS
Editors

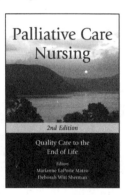

"Palliative Care Nursing is a comprehensive, well-written text that is as appropriate for practicing nurses as it is for undergraduate and graduate nursing students...The editors have paid particular attention to aspects of caring for the dying that have been neglected in nursing education: holistic integrative therapies, communication, caring for families, and peri-death nursing care."
—**Oncology Nursing Forum**

About the new edition:
"These authors and the pages of this text...create the blueprint that will build the kind of care system we all wish for our loved ones."
—From the Foreword by **Betty Rolling Ferrell,** RN, PhD, FAAN

Partial Contents:

Section I: Looking at the Whole Person in Palliative Care • Spirituality and Culture as Domains of Quality Palliative Care • Holistic Integrative Therapies in Palliative Care

Section II: Palliative Care, Society, and the Health Profession • Death and Society • Professional Organizations and Certification in Hospice and Palliative Care Nursing • The Nurse's Role as a Member of the Interdisciplinary Palliative Care Team • Ethical Aspects of Palliative Care • Legal Aspects of End-of-Life Care

Section III: Psychological Aspects of Death and Dying • Communication with Seriously Ill and Dying Patients, Their Families, and Their Health Care Providers

Section IV: Physical Aspects of Dying • Symptom Management in Palliative Care • Pain Assessment and Pharmacologic Interventions

2005 · 400pp · 978-0-8261-5794-2 · hardcover